T0214005

So-Called Alternative Medicine (SCAM) for Cancer

Edzard Ernst

So-Called Alternative Medicine (SCAM) for Cancer

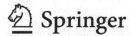 Springer

Edzard Ernst
University of Exeter
Cambridge, UK

ISBN 978-3-030-74160-0   ISBN 978-3-030-74158-7   (eBook)
https://doi.org/10.1007/978-3-030-74158-7

Thumbs symbols used in tables: © ii-graphics / stock.adobe.com

This Springer imprint is published by the registered company Springer Nature Switzerland AG
The registered company address is: Gewerbestrasse 11, 6330 Cham, Switzerland

To Danielle and Dr. Jacquot who saved her life

Foreword

In the doldrums between Christmas and New Year's Eve 2020, I was admitted to the Royal Free Hospital (RFH) in north-west London, following a heart attack. This was at the apogee of the worst pandemic in our living memory. I felt safe entering this hotbed of COVID-19, thanks to the first shot of the Pfizer vaccine two weeks before the event. Although I had once been Professor of Surgery at the RFH, I did not expect, nor was I offered, preferential treatment. I simply placed my life in the hands of our wonderful National Health Service (NHS) and went with the flow.

I was awake but sedated as they carried out my angiogram, threading a cannula up my left radial artery. The cardiologist swiftly identified the stenosis and dilated it up and cleaned out the clot. This was all done so competently, with speed and fluency, so as to minimise the damage to my myocardium (heart muscle). I marvelled at the way a cannula was navigated up my radial artery and manoeuvred into the coronary arteries on a big screen of magnified digital images. Before this intervention, my life was hanging on the threads of collateral vessels, but once unblocked, the beautiful fractal geometry of my coronary arterial system was displayed in front of my eyes and my fear was expunged. The external and internal structures of the human body are sublime, and the role of scientific medicine, aided by biotechnology of near-magical proportions, restores our bodies to functional perfection that has emerged over millions of years, through the process of evolution.

Whilst under sedation, I was in an almost transcendental state so that in my imagination I saw a long line of scientists from William Harvey who described the circulation of the blood in seventeenth century; Edward Jenner who carried the first vaccination; Louis Pasteur, without whose discoveries we would not enjoy aseptic surgery; Claude Bernard in nineteenth century who perfected out knowledge of the physiology of the cardio-vascular system; Marie Curie who won the Nobel Prize for discovering radiation at the turn of the twentieth century; Cournand, Forssmann, and Richards who shared the Nobel Prize in Physiology or Medicine in 1956; and finally the scientists Ugur Sahin and Ozlem Tureci who developed and trialled the first vaccine for the COVID-19 in record time, smiling down on me. These are just a few names of those who made the discoveries over the last 300 years that on aggregate saved my life. No thanks whatsoever to the proponents of so-called alternative medicine (SCAM), you might even go so far as to suggest that all these advances were in spite of the efforts of SCAM. We witness the worst examples of those who live in the parallel universe of the SCAMERS who spread conspiracy theories about vaccination not only for the MMR but amongst the refuseniks of the anti-COVID-19 vaccines.

This book of course is about cancer not heart disease, but my personal experience of what the NHS can achieve via evidence-based medicine (EBM), by the underlying principles, remains the same as those expressed in my personal anecdote.

I spent most of my professional life as a surgical oncologist with a specialist interest in the research and treatment of breast cancer. My interest in SCAM began in unusual circumstances nearly 40 years ago. I had recently been appointed as Professor of Surgery at Kings College London, and one of my first achievements was to raise the funds to establish a clinical trials centre for testing cancer treatments in randomised controlled trials (RCTs) throughout our Kingdom and later on to include Europe, the Common-wealth and Europe. One evening, I was invited to join in a late-night chat programme in a debate with a homeopathic doctor. At that time, I had only the vaguest ideas of what homeopathy was. Like most of my friends, I thought it was something like herbal remedies. I spoke about the progress with breast-conserving surgery and adjuvant tamoxifen that improves 10-year survival by >30% in return the homeopath lauded the success of *viscum album* also known as *Iscador*. I had no idea what that was, so he explained to me in a patronising way that it was an extract of mistletoe. When I asked how it worked in curing breast cancer, he explained to as if I was a child that mistletoe grows on oak trees like cancer grows on women; *ergo*, a *dilute* extract of *Iscador* must be good for breast cancer and that he had many anecdotes to prove this.

I could not believe my ears and made a promise to myself to research this area of ignorance. I started reading around the subject and could barely believe the nonsense in front of my eyes. By *a dilute extract* , he was describing infinitesimal dilutions wherein there was not a singular molecule of the "mother tincture" left. The choice of the "mother tincture" was based on the principle of like cures like. The simplest example might be a cure for the common cold using a very dilute extract of onion on the premise that onions make your eyes and nose run with tears and snot.

To my dismay, I learnt that there was a hospital specialising in homeopathy in London with a royal seal of approval. Royal London Homeopathic Hospital was established in 1849. It moved to its present site in Great Ormond Street in 1859. The hospital joined the NHS as a teaching hospital becoming the Royal London Homeopathic Hospital by permission of King George VI in 1948. It stopped providing NHS-funded homeopathic remedies as recently as April 2018.

Why was a bizarre blend of alternative medicine that was "invented" by an obscure German doctor in the mid-nineteenth century, the age before the enlightenment of the evidence-based medicine (EBM) era, be so popular amongst the great and the good attending a hospital with a royal warrant?

"Put not your trust in princes" (Psalm 146:3)
For reasons obscure to me, there has long been the tradition of "celebrity" endorsement.

Prominent amongst them have been Steve Jobs, Farrah Fawcett, Gwyneth Paltrow, Oprah Winfrey, Elle Macpherson, Kate Moss, Richard Gere, and Steve McQueen. Steve Jobs, the man responsible for my Apple Mac desktop upon which I type this very piece, died with pancreatic cancer. He delayed therapy for 9 months whilst searching for "natural" remedies.

Whether or not his delay influenced the outcome will never be known, but this kind of highly publicised endorsement could easily distract naïve patients with curable cancer and deny themselves the chance.

In my experience, the most alarming influencer for the promotion of alternative medicine is HRH, Prince Charles, Prince of Wales. I am guilty of Lèse-majesté by calling him to account on two occasions after his speeches at the 150th anniversary of the BMA and the bicentenary of the Royal Society. Here is an extract from an open letter I wrote at the invitation of the editor of the BMJ in 2004 [1]

Over the last 20 years, I have treated thousands of patients with cancer and lost some dear friends and relatives along the way with this dreaded disease. I guess that for the majority of my patients their first meeting with me was as momentous and memorable as mine was with you. Sadly, however hard I try, many of these courageous men and women are not instantly recognised, and covertly, I check their notes before each follow-up in order to practise the benign deception of greeting them like long lost friends. This phenomenon of asymmetrical relationships I like to describe as the "gradient of power". The power of my authority comes with a knowledge built on 40 years of study and 25 years of active involvement in cancer research. I am sensitive to the danger of abusing this power, and as a last resort, I know that the General Medical Council (GMC) is watching over my shoulder to ensure I respect a code of conduct with a duty of care that respects patient's dignity and privacy and reminds me that my personal beliefs should not prejudice my advice. If you will forgive me sir, your power and authority rests on an accident of birth. There is no equivalent of the GMC for the monarchy, so it is left to either sensational journalist or more rarely the quiet voice of loyal subject such as me, to warn you that you may have overstepped the mark. It is in the nature of your world to be surrounded by sycophants (including members of the medical establishment hungry for their mention in the Queen's birthday honours list) who constantly reinforce what they assume are your prejudices. Sir, they patronise you! Allow me this chastisement. Many lay people such as yourself have an impressionistic notion of science as a cloak for bigotry. Nothing could be further from the truth.

Professional development is part of our student's core curriculum, involving modules in the humanities. Students are taught the importance of the spiritual domain but at the same time study the epistemology of medicine, or in simpler words the nature of evidence. The scientific method is based on the deductive process that starts with the humble assumption that your hypothesis might be wrong and is then subjected to experiments that carry the risk of falsification. This approach works. For example, in my own specialist disease, breast cancer, we have witnessed a 30% fall in mortality since 1984, resulting from a world-wide collaboration in clinical trials, accompanied by improvements in quality of life as measured by psychometric instruments. You promote the Gerson diet whose only support comes from anecdotes. I have Gerson's book on my desk as I write. Forget the implausible rationale simply search for anything other than testimonial support. What is wrong with anecdote you may ask? After all, these are real human-interest stories. The problems are manifold but start with the assumption that cancer has a predictable natural history. "The patient was only given 6 months to live, tried the diet and lived for years". This is an urban myth. None of us is so arrogant as to predict that which is known only to the Almighty. With advanced breast cancer, the median expectation of life might be 18 months, but many of my patients live for many years longer, with or without treatment. I have always advocated the scientific evaluation of complementary and alternative medicine, using controlled trials, and if "alternative" therapies pass these rigorous tests of so-called orthodox" medicine, then they will cease to be alternative and join our armamentarium. If their proponents lack the courage of their convictions to have their pet remedies subjected to the "hazards of refutation", then they are the bigots who will forever be condemned to practice on the fringe. I have much time for complimentary therapy that offers improvements in quality of life or spiritual solace, providing that it is truly integrated with modern medicine, but I have no time at all for "alternative" therapy which places itself above the laws of evidence and practices in a metaphysical domain that harks back to the dark days of Galen.

Supportive treatment that complements conventional cancer medicine. As stated above, I believe there is such a concept of complementary therapy aimed at improvement in quality of life or spiritual solace and I am delighted to note that this domain is covered in a large section of this book. Unfortunately, the area of debate often gets stuck in a quagmire of semantics. In 2005, I found myself chairing a conference on the role of complementary and alternative medicine in the management of early breast cancer in Florence. [2] Professor Ernst, the author of this book, acted as a co-chairman, and I am sure he will never forget that first session where we tried to pin down the proponents of SCAM on the meaning of the words they used. Sadly, we wasted the first half day of the meeting not able to agree on the meaning of words like "complementary" and "alternative", and I suspect that the acronym SCAM, he invented, might have been germinated in Florence in 2005.

The English language has a rich and beautiful vocabulary. All these wonderful words have precise meaning, and we tamper with them at our peril. George Orwell's terrifying book 1984 illustrates the ultimate triumph of the evil of a totalitarian state. By the simple device of distorting the language as to make it impossible to even harbour subversive thoughts, "Big Brother" ruled absolutely. It saddens me to witness how the language is being debased by a pseudo-culture that encourages transient values and transient meanings to our vocabulary. The same worry concerns the use of the three words, alternative, complementary, and holistic, when applied to the practice of medicine.

The first question you have to ask about "alternative" is—alternative to what? Proponents of alternative medicine will describe the practice of doctors in the National Health Services, both in primary and tertiary care, as "orthodox", "mainstream", "Western", "reductionist", and so on. In return, the practitioners of conventional medicine view "alternative/unconventional" medicine as a series of comprehensive health belief systems, superficially with little in common, yet sharing beliefs in metaphysical concepts of balance and similarities which date back to Galenic doctrine from the second century A.D, or oriental mysticism 2,000 years older. So, in this parallel universe of alternative medicine, treatments are based on metaphysical concepts, rather than orthodox physiology and biochemistry. Yet, it has to be accepted that each view of the other is to some extent pejorative, and if we are to establish a dialogue between the champions on either side of this conceptual divide, we must show mutual trust and mutual respect. Perhaps for the time being, we might blur these distinctions by using the word "unproven" which can apply equally well to therapeutic interventions on each side. Of course, the issue of the definition of "proof" then raises problems that I will address later.

Next, we must consider the definition of "complementary". The Oxford English dictionary defines the word as, "that which completes or makes perfect, or that which when added completes a whole". In other words, whilst modern medical science struggles to cure patients, complementary medicine helps patients to feel better, and who knows, by feeling better the act of healing itself may be complemented. Some complementary approaches may be placebos, and the touch of the "healer" or the hand of the massage therapist could be guided by strange belief systems that are alien to modern science. Providing the intention is to support the clinician in his endeavours rather than compete in the relativistic marketplace of ideas one might set aside these concerns.

Finally, "holism", a slippery word whose ownership is competed for by both sides of the therapeutic divide. The word, holism, was coined by General Jan Smuts in 1926. He used the word to describe the tendency in nature to produce wholes from the ordered grouping of units (holons). Chambers twentieth-century dictionary describes holism in a precise and economic way as follows "Complete and self-contained systems from the atom and the cell by evolution to the most complex forms of life and mind". It can be perceived then that the concept of holism is complex and exquisite and as an open system lends itself to study and experimentation. As such, it should be a concept that unites us rather than a continuing source of dispute. To do justice to the definition of the word holism, we have to start at the molecular level, and then from these basic building blocks attempt to reconstruct the complex organism which is the human subject living in harmony within the complex structure of a modern democratic nation state.

The basic building block of life has to be a sequence of DNA that codes for a specific protein. These DNA sequences or genes are organised within chromosomes forming the human genome. The chromosomes are packed within the nucleus with a degree of miniaturisation, which is awe-inspiring. The nucleus is a holon looking inwards at the genome and outwards at the cytoplasm of the cell. The cell is a holon that looks inwards at the proteins, which guarantee its structure and function contained within its plasma membrane, and at the energy transduction pathways contained within the mitochondria, which produce the fuel for life. As a holon, the cell looks outwards at neighbouring cells of a self-similar type which may group together as glandular elements, but the cellular holon also enjoys cross talk with cells of a different developmental origin. These glandular elements group together as a functioning organ which is holistic in looking inwards at the exquisite functional integrity of itself and outwards to act in concert with the other organs of the body. This concert is orchestrated at the next level in the holistic hierarchy through the neuro-endocrine and immunological control mediated via the hypothalamic pituitary axis, the thyroid gland, the adrenal gland, the endocrine glands of sexual identity, and the lympho-reticular system that can distinguish self from non-self. Even this notion of "selfness" (essential individuality) is primitive compared with the next level up the hierarchy where the person exists in a conscious state somewhere within the cerebral cortex, with the mind, the great unexplored frontier, which will be the scientific challenge of doctors in the new millennium. Beyond the mind, those of strong religious faith believe in "the soul". If these religious beliefs provide solace when facing an existential crisis, then I believe it is the role of the doctors administering to the dying to enable visits from the clergy to comfort their passing.

January 2021   Prof. Michael Baum, ChM, MD, FRCS
                        Professor Emeritus of Surgery and Visiting
                        Professor of Medical Humanities, University
                        College London, London, UK

References

An open letter to the Prince of Wales: with respect, your highness, you've got it wrong BMJ 2004;329:118

Baum M, Cassileth BR, Daniel R, Ernst E, et al. The role of complementary and alternative medicine in the management of early breast cancer: recommendations of the European Society of Mastology (EUSOMA)

Eur J Cancer. 2006 Aug;42(12):1711-4

Contents

1

Introduction

1.1 Preface

In February 2013, my wife and I were in good spirits. I had recently retired from my post at Exeter University, and we were heading off to celebrate Danielle's round birthday with her family in Brittany. There was just one thing that bothered us: Danielle had recurring abdominal pains. She had seen our GP in England several times about it. The last time, she had received a prescription for some antibiotics. I knew they would not help; her symptoms were not due to an infection.

After our arrival in France, things got worse, and Danielle consulted a gynaecologist at the out-patient clinic of the local hospital. More tests were ordered; an ultrasound showed an abnormality; a subsequent MRI revealed a tumour of the uterus. The gynaecologist advised to operate as soon as possible, and Danielle agreed.

The operation went well, but the gynaecologist, Dr Matthieu Jacquot, was concerned and said he had to be more radical than he had anticipated. The diagnosis was still uncertain until the results from the histology lab were in. A few days later, when we saw Dr Jacquot again, our hopes that all was fine were thoroughly dashed. He explained that Danielle had cancer of the endometrium and laid out the treatment plan which an entire team of oncologists had designed after an in-depth review of her case: a second, much more extensive operation, followed by six sessions of chemotherapy, followed by months of daily radiotherapy, followed by two sessions of brachytherapy.

© The Author(s), under exclusive license to Springer Nature Switzerland AG 2021
E. Ernst, *So-Called Alternative Medicine (SCAM) for Cancer*,
https://doi.org/10.1007/978-3-030-74158-7_1

Dr Jacquot could not have been more empathetic. He explained in detail what consequences all this would have. Danielle's life would be dominated for the next year by a long series of treatments that were unpleasant, to say the least. We were both shocked and close to tears.

Before arriving at a decision, we talked to friends and experts in this area. Opinions differed marginally. Two days later, we had made up her mind: we would stay in Brittany for the entire year and get Danielle treated exactly as Dr Jacquot suggested.

The second operation was much tougher than the first, but Danielle recovered well. Ten days later, she was back in our home and looked after by a nurse who came daily to change the bandages and give injections. On her third visit, the nurse broached the subject of chemotherapy which was scheduled to start soon. She explained how unpleasant it would be and what horrendous side effects Danielle was facing. Then she said: 'You know, you don't need to go through all this. They only pump you full with poison. There is a much better approach. Just follow the anti-cancer diet of Dr Schwartz.[1] It is natural and has no side effects. It would surely cure your cancer.' When Danielle told me about this conversation, I informed the nurse that from now on I would myself take charge of the post-operative care of my wife and that her services were no longer required.

Today, Danielle is cancer-free. Had she listened to the nurse, she would almost certainly no longer be with us. But the lure of a 'natural' cancer cure with no side effects is almost irresistible. Faced with a serious diagnosis like cancer, most patients would consider any therapy that promises help without harm. Inevitably, they encounter a myriad of so-called alternative medicines (SCAMs), and many patients give SCAM a try.

In addition to Dr Schwartz's cancer diet, there are hundreds of SCAMs that specifically target vulnerable cancer patients like Danielle. How can patients not be confused, and who might give them responsible advice? Conventional doctors rarely do. A recent summary of 29 relevant papers concluded that *physicians will discuss complementary therapies only when a patient him/herself raises this issue within a consultation.*[2] But cancer patients are often too embarrassed to ask about SCAM. Those who are courageous enough usually get

---

[1] Dr Laurent Schwartz cancérologue iconoclaste—Guérir du Cancer (guerir-du-cancer.fr).

[2] Stub T, Quandt SA, Arcury TA, et al. Perception of risk and communication among conventional and complementary health care providers involving cancer patients' use of complementary therapies: a literature review. BMC Complement Altern Med. 2016;16(1):353. Published 2016 Sep 8. https://doi.org/10.1186/s12906-016-1326-3.

short shrift. Many conventional doctors are not just critical about SCAM, but also know very little about the subject.[3]

Patients deserve evidence-based information, instead they often get unhelpful blanket statements from their GPs such as:

- 'there is no evidence';
- 'that's all rubbish, best to stay well clear of it';
- 'if you want to try it, go ahead, it cannot do much harm'.

All of these are untrue. Frustrated by such erroneous platitudes, patients might go on the Internet for help where they are bombarded with uncritical promotion. My team investigated the information on SCAM for cancer provided by popular websites and found that they *offer information of extremely variable quality. Many endorse unproven therapies and some are outright dangerous.*[4] Sadly, the advice patients might glean from newspapers[5] or health-food stores[6] tends to be equally misleading and potentially harmful.

Subsequently, some patients might visit a library and read one of the many books on the subject. If anything, they are even worse. We have repeatedly analysed the contents of consumer guides on SCAM and always concluded that following their recommendations would shorten the life of the reader.[7] To give you a flavour, here are a few titles currently on sale:

- Cancer Medicine from Nature
- Outsmart Your Cancer: Alternative Non-Toxic Treatments That Work
- Cancer Medicine from Nature
- Perfect Guide on How to Cure Breast Cancer Through Curative Approved Alkaline Diets & Herbs
- How to Starve Cancer
- Healing the Prostate: The Best Holistic Methods to Treat the Prostate and Other Common Male-Related Conditions

---

[3] Ziodeen KA, Misra SM. Complementary and integrative medicine attitudes and perceived knowledge in a large pediatric residency program. *Complement Ther Med*. 2018;37:133–135. https://doi.org/10.1016/j.ctim.2018.02.004.

[4] Schmidt K, Ernst E. Assessing websites on complementary and alternative medicine for cancer. *Ann Oncol*. 2004;15(5):733–742. https://doi.org/10.1093/annonc/mdh174.

[5] Milazzo S, Ernst E. Newspaper coverage of complementary and alternative therapies for cancer–UK 2002–2004. *Support Care Cancer*. 2006;14(9):885–889. https://doi.org/10.1007/s00520-006-0068-z

[6] Mills E, Ernst E, Singh R, Ross C, Wilson K. Health food store recommendations: implications for breast cancer patients. *Breast Cancer Res*. 2003;5(6):R170-R174. https://doi.org/10.1186/bcr636.

[7] https://edzardernst.com/2013/09/drowning-in-a-sea-of-misinformation-part-8-books-on-alternative-medicine/.

- Outsmart Cancer: Defeat Cancer With Vitamin B17, Healthy Nutrition and Alternative Medicine.

Cancer patients would, of course, all like to 'outsmart cancer'; they are desperate and vulnerable. In this state of mind, they easily fall victim to anyone who sells false hope at inflated prices. The consequences can be tragic.

In 2016, the actress English Leah Bracknell, for example, raised ~ £50,000 to treat her lung cancer in the 'Hallwang Private Oncology Clinic' in Germany. The SCAMs used there included homoeopathy, micronutrients, natural supplements, whole-body hyperthermia and ozone therapy, none of which cures cancer. If cancer patients fall for bogus treatments, they not just lose their money but also their lives. Leah Bracknell died of her cancer in 2019.[8]

Three basic facts indisputably clear:

- a high percentage of cancer patients use SCAM,
- misinformation about SCAM is rife,
- misinformation endangers the lives of cancer patients.

It follows that there is an obvious and urgent need for an evidence-based text naming the SCAMs that are potentially harmful and discussing those that might be helpful.

This book is aimed at doing just that.

1.2   Definition of SCAM and Related Terms

We used to call it 'alternative medicine', the name most people still know best. But lately, I have started employing a different term for it; I now tend to call it **so-called alternative medicine** or **SCAM** for short.

Why?

Mainly because, whatever it is, it clearly is not an alternative:

- If therapy does <u>not</u> work, it cannot possibly be a reasonable alternative to an effective treatment.
- And if it <u>does</u> work, it simply is part of medicine.

---

[8] https://edzardernst.com/2019/10/leah-blacknell-1964-2019-another-victim-of-cancer-quackery/.

After having been involved in this subject for over 25 years, I feel that 'SCAM' is preferable to the many vague and imprecise terms that have been used previously:

- ALTERNATIVE MEDICINE describes therapeutic and diagnostic modalities employed as a replacement for conventional modalities.
- COMPLEMENTARY MEDICINE is an umbrella term for modalities usually employed as an adjunct to conventional healthcare.
- COMPLEMENTARY AND ALTERNATIVE MEDICINE (CAM) combines both expressions acknowledging that the same modality is often employed either as a replacement for or an add-on to conventional medicine.
- DISPROVEN MEDICINE is an umbrella term for treatments that have been tested and shown not to work.
- FRINGE MEDICINE is a derogatory term no longer used.
- HOLISTIC MEDICINE is healthcare that emphasises whole patient care.
- INTEGRATIVE MEDICINE allegedly incorporates 'the best of both worlds', i.e. the best of SCAM and conventional healthcare.
- NATURAL MEDICINE is healthcare exclusively relying on the means provided by nature.
- TRADITIONAL MEDICINE is healthcare that has been in use for a long time and is thus assumed to have stood the test of time.
- UNCONVENTIONAL MEDICINE is healthcare not normally used in conventional medicine (this would include off-label use of drugs, for instance, and therefore is not an appropriate term for SCAM).
- UNORTHODOX MEDICINE is a term for healthcare that is not normally used in orthodox medicine.
- UNPROVEN MEDICINE is healthcare that lacks scientific proof (many conventional therapies also fall in this category too).

And how do I define SCAM? The way I see it, **SCAM is an umbrella term for many therapeutic and a few diagnostic modalities that are not generally accepted as useful by conventional healthcare professionals while being promoted as helpful by practitioners operating outside the mainstream of medicine.**

One obstacle to finding a suitable name is, of course, that SCAM includes a wide range of highly diverse modalities (in a recent book,[9] I evaluated 150,

---

[9] Alternative Medicine: A Critical Assessment of 150 Modalities: Amazon.co.uk: Ernst, Edzard: Books.

but in total there are well over 400 in total) that do not easily fit under one single umbrella. Some of the most popular therapies include:

- **Acupuncture** involves the insertion of needles into the skin and underlying tissues at acupuncture points for therapeutic or preventative purposes (Sect. 4.1).
- **Anthroposophic medicine** is based on the mystical concepts of Rudolf Steiner. Various treatments are employed by anthroposophic doctors, the most famous of which is mistletoe (Sect. 3.1).
- **Aromatherapy** employs 'essential' oils usually combined with gentle massage; less commonly the oils are applied via inhalation (Sect. 4.2).
- **Chiropractic** is a SCAM that was developed about 120 years ago by DD Palmer. The hallmark therapy of chiropractors is spinal manipulation which, they claim, is necessary to adjust 'subluxations' (Sect. 4.7).
- **Crystal healing** uses the alleged power of crystals to stimulate the self-healing properties of the body (Sect. 4.6).
- **Dietary supplements** are preparations intended to supplement the diet; they can contain vitamins, minerals, herbal remedies and other substances (Sects. 3.1, 3.4, 4.4, 4.5).
- **Energy or paranormal healing** are umbrella terms for several SCAMs that rely on the use of 'energy' or vital force (Sect. 4.6).
- **Herbal medicine** (or phytotherapy) is the medicinal use of preparations that exclusively contain plant material (Sects. 3.1, 4.4).
- **Homoeopathy** is a therapeutic method using substances whose effects, when administered to healthy subjects, correspond to the manifestations of the disorder in the individual patient (Sect. 3.2).
- **Mind–body therapies** are SCAMs which are thought to influence bodily functions via the mind (Sect. 4.3).
- **Naturopathy** is a type of healthcare that employs what nature provides (e. g. herbal extracts, manual therapies, heat and cold, water and electricity) for stimulating the body's ability to heal itself (Sect. 4.7).
- **Osteopathy** is a manual therapy involving manipulation of the spine and other joints as well as mobilization of soft tissues (Sect. 4.7).
- **Reflexology** is a SCAM employing manual pressure to specific areas of the body, usually the feet, which are claimed to correspond to internal organs with a view of generating positive health effects (Sect. 4.2).
- **Reiki** is a Japanese SCAM where the therapist claims to channel vital energy into the patient's body, a process that allegedly stimulates his self-healing abilities (Sect. 4.6).

- **Therapeutic Touch** is a form of energy healing where the therapist claims to channel life energy into the patient's body which is said to stimulate his/her self-healing abilities (Sect. 4.6).
- **Traditional Chinese Medicine** is a diagnostic and therapeutic system based on the Taoist philosophy of Yin and Yang. It includes SCAMs like acupuncture, herbal medicine, tui-na (Chinese massage), tai chi and diet (Sects. 3.1, 4.1, 4.2).

In recent decades, these therapies have become important, not least because large proportions (25% (UK)—70% (Germany)) of the general population use them. Cancer patients, in particular, can hardly ignore the relentless promotion of SCAM. The usage of SCAM can therefore be even higher in cancer victims than in the general population. A 2012 summary of studies from 18 countries showed that the average use of SCAM by cancer patients was 40%.[10] The financial burden caused by SCAM use can be considerable.[11] The reasons for SCAM's popularity are complex; they vary according to the type of SCAM, and differ from one individual to another. For cancer patients, some of the main motivations for trying SCAM include,[12,13]:

- the wish to try everything that promises a cure,
- the disappointment with conventional oncology,
- the hope for a risk-free treatment,
- the fear of the adverse effects of conventional treatments,
- the hope to reduce the side effects of conventional treatments,
- the wish to improve quality of life,
- the hope to be able to cope better during difficult times.

---

[10] Horneber M, Bueschel G, Dennert G, Less D, Ritter E, Zwahlen M. How many cancer patients use complementary and alternative medicine: a systematic review and metaanalysis. Integr Cancer Ther. 2012 Sep;11(3):187–203. https://doi.org/10.1177/1534735411423920. Epub 2011 Oct 21. PMID: 22019489.

[11] Longo CJ, Fitch MI, Loree JM, Carlson LE, Turner D, Cheung WY, Gopaul D, Ellis J, Ringash J, Mathews M, Wright J, Stevens C, D'Souza D, Urquhart R, Maity T, Balderrama F, Haddad E. Patient and family financial burden associated with cancer treatment in Canada: a national study. Support Care Cancer. 2021 Jan 5. https://doi.org/10.1007/s00520-020-05907-x. Epub ahead of print. PMID: 33403399.

[12] Ernst E. Alternative treatments for breast cancer. *Eur J Clin Pharmacol*. 2012;68(5):453–454. https://doi.org/10.1007/s00228-011-1186-1

[13] Tangkiatkumjai M, Boardman H, Walker DM. Potential factors that influence usage of complementary and alternative medicine worldwide: a systematic review. BMC Complement Med Ther. 2020 Nov 23;20(1):363. https://doi.org/10.1186/s12906-020-03157-2. PMID: 33228697; PMCID: PMC7686746.

These motivations also suggest that cancer patients who decide to try SCAM are guided by certain assumptions. The next chapter will discuss some of these notions and ask whether they are realistic.

1.3   Common Assumptions About SCAM

Even though SCAM is a confusingly diverse area, there are some general assumptions that are often made for it. In this chapter, I will discuss some of the notions that seem important in the context of this book and explain how they are often used to mislead cancer patients.

SCAM Is Helpful

Cancer patients who try SCAM evidently hope that they will benefit from it. We will discuss the scientific evidence for specific therapies in Chaps. 2, 3 and 4 of this book. Suffice to say that the assumption of effectiveness is by no means always correct. Often it is a true leap of faith, and patients who make this leap blindly might pay dearly for their error.

A prominent example is Steve Jobs, the co-founder of Apple computers. Assuming that SCAM is effective, he delayed using conventional treatments for his pancreatic cancer. Based on the advice from SCAM practitioners, he decided to employ various SCAMs instead. When Jobs finally realised that he had made a mistake, it was too late and he died only months later. *Steve Jobs' decision to try an unproven therapeutic approach in the face of medical uncertainly was no different from similar decisions routinely made by many cancer patients. Jobs' example teaches that even those individuals with access to the most resources cannot make informed decisions about the use of conventional and/or CAM therapies if the information does not exist.*[14]

This and many similarly tragic cases serve as a powerful reminder of how risky erroneous assumptions about SCAM can be. Wishful thinking is only human but, in the realm of healthcare, it is certainly no substitute for reliable evidence.

---

[14] Greenlee H, Ernst E. What can we learn from Steve Jobs about complementary and alternative therapies?. *Prev Med*. 2012;54(1):3–4. https://doi.org/10.1016/j.ypmed.2011.12.014

SCAM Is Natural and Therefore Safe

Few qualities attract consumers more than the claim of being natural. A multi-billion-dollar industry has thus developed around the assertion that SCAM is natural. At first glance, it seems that many forms of SCAM are indeed entirely natural:

- acupuncture is perceived as natural;
- essential oils are perceived as natural;
- herbal remedies are perceived as natural;
- homeopathy is perceived as natural;
- naturopathy even derives its name from being natural
- etc., etc.

In fact, it is hard to think of a SCAM that is not being promoted as natural. But, if we think critically about such assumptions, we find that there is nothing natural about SCAMs:

- acupuncture involves the unnatural process of sticking needles into the skin of a patient;
- essential oils are distilled and unnaturally concentrated volatile substances;
- herbal supplements are often highly processed;
- homeopathy employs artificial materials like, for instance, the Berlin wall;
- naturopaths use all sorts of unnatural procedures such as neural therapy (injection of a local anaesthetic), for instance.

We automatically assume that natural treatments generate more good than harm. Somehow, we seem to be hard-wired to think that mother nature is always benign. Apt examples are the many books for cancer victims that use 'natural' in their title:

A book entitled *Cancer: Natural cures they don't want you to know about*[15] is being advertised with the following text:
This book will offer you other natural alternative ways that will help you fight your illness. Cancer: Natural Cures "That they don't want you to know about" will help you understand: • *How to beat cancer by rebalancing your bodies pH back to a normal level* • *Natural Cures that have helped save the lives of thousands at any stage of cancer* • *Understanding what feeds cancer and makes it grow* • *Simple*

---

[15] https://www.amazon.co.uk/Cancer-Natural-Cures-They-about/dp/1490905790.

*testing that allows you to know if you still have cancer cells within your body •
Starving cancer cells by the intake of nutrition and supplements and much more.
Once you have the proper understanding and education of the cause of your cancer,
you can beat anything with your mind, body and spirit! It's time to take charge of
your life because no one else is going to do it for you.*

A book entitled *Gentle Cures For Tough Cancers. Non-Toxic, God-Given
Natural Cures That Work*[16] tempts patients with this advertisement:

*… this new book … describes the best and most effective natural cures for
fighting cancer. Have you or someone you love been diagnosed with cancer and told
that chemo and radiation are your only hope? Gentle Cures contains true stories of
cancer victims, who were told they were dying, yet they are still alive and well, years
later, after using non-toxic treatments described in this book. You will read about
new cancer tests, safer drugs and gentler treatments now available. There are many
new drugs, described in this book, that are not even called "chemo" drugs because
they are non-toxic. You will find that healing involves the mind, body and soul,
and the importance of prayer in approaching God for healing yourself and those
you love. You will also read many helpful tips for fighting M.S., arthritis, asthma,
allergies, colon problems, COPD, migraines, hepatitis and other health disorders.*

Another book is bluntly entitled *Natural Cancer Cures*[17] and informs us
that *cancer is caused by deoxygenation of cells and infection, and it can be cured.
This book explains how cancer onsets within the human body; and how it can be
reversed into complete remission.*

These examples highlight several important points:

1. The term 'natural' is a popular marketing tool for the promotion of
   SCAMs.
2. Proponents of SCAM often have bizarre ideas about cancer.
3. Practitioners of SCAM tend to discourage the use of effective conventional
   treatments.
4. Proponents of SCAM like to disguise anecdotes as evidence.
5. Promoters of SCAM endanger the life of cancer patients who follow their
   absurd advice.

The disappointing truth is that SCAM has few qualities that would truly
render it natural. And, of course, natural does not necessarily mean harmless—think of a tornado, lightening, infections, hemlock, etc.; they are all as
natural as they are dangerous. As we will discuss in more detail in Sect. 1.3 of
this book, many SCAMs advertised as natural are neither effective nor safe.

---

[16] https://www.amazon.co.uk/Gentle-Cures-Tough-Cancers-Non-Toxic/dp/1603831150.
[17] https://www.goodreads.com/book/show/17927945-natural-cancer-cures.

SCAM Defies Scientific Investigation

Enthusiasts of SCAM frequently claim that the scientific method is not a tool that is applicable to their field. Several reasons are offered for this notion, e.g.:

- The effects of SCAM are too subtle to be quantified with the blunt instruments of science.
- SCAMs need to be tailored to each individual and therefore they cannot be submitted to testing in clinical trials.
- The therapeutic approach of SCAM is holistic (see below), which means it cannot be evaluated with reductionistic science.

These claims might convince consumers who already are believers in SCAM; however, on closer inspection, they turn out to be false. As we will discuss later, they are either based on deliberate attempts to deceive or on profound misunderstandings of what science in general and the clinical trial in particular can achieve (Sect. 1.8).

Rather than addressing these issues in detail, it may suffice to point out that SCAM proponents do enthusiastically accept scientific investigations of their intervention—as long as their results are positive. There are now thousands of clinical trials of SCAM, many of which suggest that some SCAM interventions do generate more good than harm (see Sect. 1.4 of this book). In these instances, SCAM enthusiasts seem to quickly forget their objections to rigorous science.

The 'Establishment' Wants to Suppress SCAM

Proponents of SCAM often claim that they and their treatments are the victims of a well-coordinated attack by 'big pharma', 'the scientific establishment' or some other sinister organisation. They seem to believe that dark forces are secretly at work aiming to prevent cancer patients from benefiting from SCAM. Essentially, this notion suggests that oncologists are a malign clique of conspirators who would withhold effective treatments from suffering cancer patients for the sole reason that they were developed or discovered by people who do not belong to their profession.

The popularity of this argument contrasts sharply with the void of evidence that it is true. In the many years of researching this area, I have never come across any evidence for the notion that SCAM is being suppressed by 'Big Pharma' or anyone else. On the contrary, as soon as this looks profitable, the pharmaceutical industry and the medical establishment are usually keen to jump on to the alternative bandwagon and maximise their profit by selling SCAM products. Similarly, universities, hospitals, charities and other organisations in healthcare are currently bending over backwards to accommodate as much SCAM as they possibly can get away with. Whenever I asked a believer in the conspiracy theory of the suppression of SCAM to show me any evidence for his assumptions, I ended up empty-handed. There simply is no such evidence.

SCAM Is Holistic

Practitioners of SCAM are keen to point out that they practice holistic healthcare by caring for the whole person, body, mind and spirit (Sect. 1.6). Virtually every book ever published on SCAM emphasises this notion. Many SCAM practitioners even go one decisive step further by claiming to be the only clinicians who practice holistically. This has the added effect of putting patients off conventional medicine because, by implication, it is characterised as non-holistic.

This notion, however, flies in the face of known facts. Holism has always been a central element of any good healthcare. While SCAM practitioners claim to be holistic, they have at best an amateur approach of caring for the whole patient.

- They often are not adequately trained to deal with complex conditions like cancer.
- They regularly over-estimate their own ability to deal with serious conditions.
- They rarely refer their patients to other healthcare professionals.

Consequently, SCAM is usually less holistic than the practice of modern healthcare. And less holistic can also mean more dangerous. There are many cases to demonstrate this point. Here is the short summary of a particularly tragic one:

> An elderly woman with a sore throat consulted her holistic doctor homeopath. The doctor prescribed homeopathic remedies. The patient continued with this approach for months, evidently without success. Only 10 months later, she changed her doctor, and her new physician sent her straight into hospital where she was diagnosed with throat cancer. After 4 years of suffering, the woman

died.[18] Having wasted 10 months with a 'holistic' approach meant it was too late to save her life.

And why do so many SCAM practitioners claim to be holistic? The answer is simple: the claim is attractive to consumers, and consequently it is good for business.

There Is no Evidence

In discussions about SCAM, we often hear: 'There is no (or not enough) evidence for or against SCAM'. The argument can cut both ways:

- Proponents of SCAM use it to imply firstly that their field has long been neglected by 'the establishment', and secondly to claim that in the absence of evidence we must give SCAM the benefit of the doubt. As long as there is no proof that it does not work, they should be entitled to use it.
- Critics of SCAM use the argument to point out that SCAM is unproven and therefore must not be used in clinical routine.

As it turns out, both sides are wrong. A simple Medline search (Medline is the largest database for medical papers) shows that there are currently well over 300,000 published papers in the category of 'alternative medicine', about 40,000 of which seem to be clinical trials. For specific SCAMs, we also find sizeable amounts of Medline-listed publications:

- Acupuncture: ~ 33,000
- Herbal medicine: ~ 47,000
- Mind–body therapy: ~ 53,000
- Massage: ~ 17,000
- Dietary supplements: ~ 87,000

These figures are smaller than those for many areas of conventional medicine, but they are nevertheless substantial and they demonstrate that the argument 'there is no evidence' is simply not true.

As we will see in the following sections of this book, the problem with the evidence is not so much its scarcity but its quality and its direction. For some specific SCAMs used to treat cancer patients, there is enough evidence to conclude that they are worth trying (Chap. 4). But for many others,

---

[18] https://edzardernst.com/2018/05/this-is-what-happens-if-you-treat-cancer-with-homeopathy/.

the evidence fails to be positive in which case they can, of course, not be recommended for routine usage.

1.4   Cancer and SCAM[19]*

This short section is aimed at explaining some essential facts about cancer. It is by no means an exhaustive review of the subject but covers merely a few selected issues that seem relevant in the context of this book.

Many SCAM proponents think of cancer as one single disease. This notion is incorrect; cancer is, in fact, a group of more than hundred different diseases. They have in common that some cells of our body start dividing without the control that normally governs cell growth (experts speak of malignant cells), and that some of the out-of-control, malignant cells can migrate to distant locations in the body (experts speak of metastases). A key characteristic of malignant cells is that they also invade the surrounding or underlying tissue (this is one of the features that distinguishes a benign from a malignant tumour). Metastases are more likely as the cancer advances and they usually have a poor prognosis. This is one of the reasons why cancer should be detected early before it had time to spread. Cancers spread in three ways:

- locally, by invading surrounding structures,
- regionally, via the lymphatic vessels to lymph nodes,
- distantly, via the blood.

Metastases are secondary tumours arising from spread to lymph nodes or other organs. The lungs, liver, bones and brain are common sites of spread. The tendency to metastasise varies according to the type of the cancer.

Many theories about the origins of cancer held by proponents of SCAM are in overt conflict with our modern understanding of cancer. For instance, some believe that cancers are caused by stress or trauma, others by an imbalance of the patient's vital forces, others by energy blockages in the body, others by toxic by-products of the body's metabolism, others by a deficient immune system (a deficient immune system can, in fact, lead to malignancy. Non-Hodgkin's lymphoma is an AIDS-defining illness in an HIV-positive individual (i.e. marking the moment when HIV becomes AIDS). When proponents of SCAM talk about a deficient immune system, it is unclear

---

[19] I am grateful to Dr Julian Money-Kyrle, retired consultant oncologist, for his constructive comments on a draft version of this section.

what exactly they mean by it.). Such phenomena may be contributing or aggravating factors in certain situations, however, they are not causes of a cancer.

Some people also believe that any tumour is a cancer. Yet, the term 'tumour' merely describes a solid mass of tissue or lump. There are cancerous (malignant) tumours, benign tumours (not growing out of control), and borderline tumours which might turn malignant at a later stage or which grow so slowly that they might not be a danger to the patient's health. Benign tumours can still be fatal—for instance, a large meningioma can compress the brain and cause significant damage as there is no room inside the skull for it to grow. Although benign tumours are generally slow-growing and usually fairly harmless, the key difference between benign and malignant tumours is invasion and metastasis. And there are some cancers that do not form tumours at all, for instance, leukaemia.

We normally define cancers by the organ they originate from; common cancers are breast, prostate, lung and colon cancer. Virtually every organ of the body can develop cancer. Another way to classify cancer is according to the tissue of origin:

- Carcinomas arise from the epithelium, the cell layers that cover organs.
- Sarcomas arise from bone, muscle or blood vessel tissue (i.e. the connective tissue).
- Gliomas arise from the glial cells of the central nervous system
- Leukaemias arise from the bone marrow.
- Lymphomas arise from lymphocytes and related cells.

Low-grade tumours are generally slow-growing and late to spread; high-grade tumours may well have already spread by the time they are diagnosed. Grading is based on the microscopic appearance including such findings as to how many of the cells are in the process of dividing and how much they resemble normal cells. It is related to differentiation—well-differentiated tumours tend to be low-grade, whereas poorly-differentiated and undifferentiated tumours are high grade; the most undifferentiated tumours are referred to as anaplastic.

One of the key things that doctors treating cancer need to establish is the stage, which is a measure of how advanced the disease is and how far it has spread. Different staging systems are used for different types of cancer, but in general stage 1 refers to a small tumour that is confined to its site of origin, whereas stage 4 means that there are secondary tumours at other sites. Staging is usually established by radiographic imaging, such as CT scans, PET scans and MRI. Biopsies are required to confirm the diagnosis of cancer, to determine the type and to assess the grade.

Cancers are common diseases; about one in three women and one in two men must expect to develop a cancer during their lifetime. Most cancers become more common as we grow older. Strictly speaking, cancer is a disease of the DNA. A sequence of about six mutations occurring in the same cell is required for it to turn malignant. Sometimes a person is born with one of these mutations already present in all of their cells, in which case we say that they are carrying a cancer gene. These are often genes involved in the DNA repair mechanism, and if this is faulty then further mutations can take place more easily. More generally, people tend to resemble their parents, so even in the absence of a known cancer gene, a family history of cancer can be a risk factor. Important risk factors are tobacco, diet, alcohol, sunlight, infections, pollution, overweight and lack of physical activity. There are several early warning signs that could be indicative of a cancer developing, for instance:

- A persistent cough might be a sign of lung cancer.
- A change in the size or colour of a skin mole could be a sign of skin cancer.
- A lump in a breast might suggest breast cancer.
- A change in bowel habits could be a sign of colon cancer.
- Weight loss, fatigue or pain can be signs of several types of cancer.
- Unexplained bleeding somewhere, for instance, coughing up blood or blood in the stool or urine might be signs of cancer of the lungs, bowel or bladder.

The diagnosis of cancer relies on thorough history taking, physical examination of the patient, various imaging techniques and biopsies. This will provide the precise cancer type and stage which in turn determines the optimal therapeutic approach.

Treatment varies according to cancer type and stage and must be tailor-made to the needs of each individual patient. Research into this area is very active; consequently new therapies or treatment regimens are being developed continuously. The main options include:

- surgery,
- chemotherapy,
- targeted therapies such as monoclonal antibodies,
- radiation,
- immunotherapy,
- hormone therapy,

- bone marrow transplant,
- stem cell treatment.

All of these treatments have side effects which can be severe and impact patients' quality of life. Proponents of SCAM often focus on these adverse effects and stress that chemotherapy, for instance, is toxic and should be avoided. This argument ignores that the value of a therapy is determined by its risk/benefit balance. Conventional cancer treatments do unquestionably cause severe side effects in some cases, but they have a realistic potential to save the patient's life. Therefore, their risk/benefit balance is in most patients' estimation still positive.

It can be difficult to predict who is going to get severe side effects and who not; this can be due to individual differences in how drugs are metabolised, or how efficiently DNA is repaired following radiation damage. In order to reduce such side effects, oncologists prescribe a range of treatments. Many cancer patients also try SCAM in the hope to further reduce the adverse effects of the therapy or for enabling them to better cope with the anxieties and stress of having cancer. This will be the subject of Sect. 1.4 of this book.

The prognosis of most cancers has vastly improved during the last few decades. If caught early, many cancers are today curable. Some advanced cancers are curable too, for instance, most lymphomas and nearly all testicular cancers. Whether SCAM can change the natural history of cancer will be the subject of Sect. 1.3 of this book.

1.5 Integrative Cancer Care

Proponents claim that integrative medicine (IM) is based mainly on two concepts:

- whole person care,
- combining "the best of both worlds".

Attractive concepts, one might think, but how valid are they really?

Whole Patient Care or Holism

Integrative healthcare practitioners, we are being told, do not just treat the physical complaints of a patient but look after the whole individual: body, mind and spirit. On the surface, this approach seems most laudable. Yet a closer look reveals major problems.

As already pointed out in Sect. 1.3, good medicine is, was, and always will be holistic; and this clearly includes cancer care. Any good oncology team should care for their patients as whole individuals dealing the best they can with physical problems as well as social and spiritual issues. I said "should" because some do neglect the holistic aspect of care. If that happens, it is by definition not good healthcare. And, if the deficit is wide spread, we must reform conventional healthcare. But delegating holism to SCAM practitioners would be tantamount to abandoning an essential element of good medicine; it would be a serious disservice to today's patients and a detriment to the healthcare of tomorrow.

It follows that the promotion of integrative cancer care under the banner of holism makes little sense. It either misleads cancer patients into believing holism is an exclusive feature of IM, while, in fact, it is a hallmark of any good healthcare. Or (if holism is neglected or absent in a particular branch of conventional cancer care) it detracts us from the important task of identifying and rectifying a regrettable deficit in conventional oncology and thus prevents progress.

The Best of Both Worlds

The second concept of IM is often described as "the best of both worlds". Proponents of IM claim to use the "best" of the world of SCAM and combine it with the "best" of conventional healthcare. Again, this concept looks commendable at first glance but, at closer inspection, serious doubts emerge.

They hinge on the use of the term "best", and we have to ask, what does "best" mean in the context of healthcare? Surely it cannot mean the most popular, fashionable or politically correct. Best can only signify "the most effective" or more precisely it means those treatments that are associated with the most convincingly positive risk–benefit balance.

If we understand "the best of both worlds" in this way, the concept becomes synonymous with the concept of evidence-based medicine (EBM) which represents the accepted thinking in any healthcare, including of course oncology. According to the principles of EBM, treatments must be shown to be reasonably safe as well as effective, and doctors should combine this evidence with their own experience as well as with the preferences of their patients.

If "the best of both worlds" is synonymous with EBM, we clearly don't need this duplicity of terminology in the first place; it would only confuse and distract from the auspicious efforts of EBM to continuously improve cancer care. In other words, the second concept of IM is just as nonsensical as the first.

Yet, integrative cancer care (ICC) is currently being heavily promoted as a major advance in cancer care. Here is just one example; as it is in German, allow me to translate it for you [the numbers added to the text refer to my comments below]:

ICC is a method of treatment that views humans holistically [1]. The approach is characterised by a synergistic application (integration) of all conventional, immunological, biological and psychological insights [2]. In this spirit, also personal needs and subjective experiences of disease are accounted for [3]. The aim of this special approach is to offer cancer patients an individualised, interdisciplinary treatment [4].

Besides surgery, chemotherapy and radiotherapy, ICC also includes hormone therapy, hyperthermia, pain management, immunotherapy, normalisation of metabolism, stabilisation of the psyche, physical activity, dietary changes, as well as substitution of vital nutrients [5].

With ICC, the newest discoveries of cancer research are being offered [6], that support the aims of ICC. Therefore, the aims of the ICT doctor include continuous research of the world literature on oncology [7]...

Likewise, one has to start immediately with measures that help prevent metastases and tumour progression [8]. Both the maximisation of survival and the optimisation of quality of life ought to be guaranteed [9]. Therefore, the alleviation of the side effects of the aggressive therapies are one of the most important aims of ICC [10]...[20]

1. Actually, this describes conventional oncology!
2. Actually, this describes conventional oncology!
3. Actually, this describes conventional oncology!
4. Actually, this describes conventional oncology!
5. Actually, this describes conventional oncology!
6. Actually, this describes conventional oncology!
7. Actually, this describes conventional oncology!
8. Actually, this describes conventional oncology!
9. Actually, this describes conventional oncology!
10. Actually, this describes conventional oncology!

---

[20] I finally found out what integrative cancer therapy is ... IT'S A CONFIDENCE TRICK! (edzardernst.com).

This confirms what we discussed above: IM 'borrows' principles and concept from conventional medicine and pretends they are unique to SCAM. If that is so, IM is not a constructive addition to healthcare. Many experts agree that IM is an ill-conceived idea; for example, Canadian vascular surgeons put it succinctly[21]:

Evidence-based medicine, first described in 1992, offers a clear, systematic, and scientific approach to the practice of medicine. Recently, the non-evidence-based practice of complementary and alternative medicine (CAM) has been increasing in the United States and around the world, particularly at medical institutions known for providing rigorous evidence-based care. The use of CAM may cause harm to patients through interactions with evidence-based medications or if patients choose to forego evidence-based care. CAM may also put financial strain on patients as most CAM expenditures are paid out-of-pocket. Despite these drawbacks, patients continue to use CAM due to media promotion of CAM therapies, dissatisfaction with conventional healthcare, and a desire for more holistic care. Given the increasing demand for CAM, many medical institutions now offer CAM services. Recently, there has been controversy surrounding the leaders of several CAM centres based at a highly respected academic medical institution, as they publicly expressed anti-vaccination views. These controversies demonstrate the non-evidence-based philosophies that run deep within CAM that are contrary to the evidence-based care that academic medical institutions should provide. Although there are financial incentives for institutions to provide CAM, it is important to recognize that this legitimizes CAM and may cause harm to patients. The poor regulation of CAM allows for the continued distribution of products and services that have not been rigorously tested for safety and efficacy. Governments in Australia and England have successfully improved regulation of CAM and can serve as a model to other countries.

Integrative Medicine and Research

So, the theoretical underpinning of IM is questionable, but what about the research into this subject? In 2012, I published an analysis of the 2010 '3rd European Congress of Integrated Medicine'. For this purpose, I categorised all of the 222 published abstracts according to their subject area. The results showed that the vast majority were on unproven SCAMs and none were on

[21] Li B, Forbes TL, Byrne J. Integrative medicine or infiltrative pseudoscience? Surgeon. 2018 Oct;16(5):271–277. https://doi.org/10.1016/j.surge.2017.12.002. Epub 2018 Jan 2. PMID: 29305045.

conventional treatments.[22] The 2016 International Congress on Integrative Medicine & Health gave me the opportunity to check whether, meanwhile this situation had changed. There were around 400 abstracts, and I did essentially the same type of analysis.[23] Here are the results (the numbers in brackets signify the number of abstracts on the topic):

- mind–body therapies (49),
- acupuncture (44),
- herbal medicine (37),
- integrative medicine (36),
- chiropractic and other manual therapies (26),
- Traditional Chinese Medicine (19),
- methodological issues (16),
- animal studies and other pre-clinical investigations (15),
- Tai Chi (5).

The rest of the abstracts were on a diverse array of other subjects. There was not a single paper on conventional therapy and only four focussed on risk assessments. The majority of the 36 abstracts on IM focussed on the SCAMs in question and concluded that this 'integration' was followed by good results. None of these papers discussed the assumptions of IM critically, and none cast any doubt about the notion that IM is a good idea.

These two analyses of conference abstracts published 6 years apart, therefore, demonstrate the same phenomenon: research into IM is not at all about the 'best of both worlds'. It is almost exclusively about the world of SCAM in which advocates of IM aim to create a smokescreen behind which they can smuggle dubious treatments into conventional healthcare.

The Practice of Integrative Medicine

On the basis of these considerations, IM is a superfluous, misleading as well as counterproductive distraction, and the research into IM is of questionable value. But by far the most powerful argument against IM is an entirely practical one; it relates to the dubious things that are happening every day in its name and under its banner.

---

[22] Ernst E. Integrated medicine. *J Intern Med*. 2012;271(1):25–28. https://doi.org/10.1111/j.1365-2796.2011.02417.x.

[23] The International Congress on Integrative Medicine and Health (ICIMH), Las Vegas, Nevada, USA May 17–20, 2016. *J Altern Complement Med*. 2016;22(6):A1-A142. https://doi.org/10.1089/acm.2016.29003.abstracts.

If we look around us, go on the Internet, read the relevant literature, or walk into an IM clinic in our neighbourhood, we are bound to discover that behind the slogans of holism and "best of all worlds" lurks the ugly face of pure quackery. Perhaps you don't believe me, so please do make the effort and look for yourself. I promise you will discover any unproven and disproven therapy that you can think of, anything from crystal healing to Reiki, and from homeopathy to urine therapy. The very first clinic that I found today (2/11/2020) when googling 'integrative oncology clinic' offered many questionable modalities, including:

- homeopathy,
- iridology,
- hair analysis,
- live blood analysis.

What follows from all this is sad and simple: integrative cancer care is little more than a front of half-baked concepts that allow the application of bogus SCAMs to vulnerable cancer patients. I find it hard to think of anything less ethical than that. And the ethical issues raised by SCAM will be the subject of the next chapter.

1.6   Ethical Issues

Medical ethics comprise a set of rules and principles which are fundamental to all aspects of healthcare:

- Respect for autonomy—e.g. patients must have the right to refuse or choose their treatments.
- Beneficence—e.g. healthcare professionals must act in the best interest of the patient.
- Non-maleficence—e.g. the proven benefits of interventions must outweigh their risks.
- Justice—e.g. the distribution of health resources must be fair.
- Respect for persons—e.g. patients must be treated with dignity.
- Truthfulness and honesty—e.g. informed consent must offer full and truthful information and is an essential element both in medical research and clinical practice.

While all of this has long been the accepted standard in conventional healthcare, it often seems flagrantly neglected in SCAM. Therefore, it is relevant to ask, to what extent does SCAM abide by the rules of medical ethics? In this chapter, I will discuss merely a small selection of ethical issues that are most relevant in the context of this book (for a fuller discussion, see our recent book[24]).

Nonsensical or Wasteful Research

At best, nonsensical research is a waste of precious resources, at worst it violates the beneficence principle, as it is not in the best interest of patients and progress. In SCAM, nonsensical research occurs with lamentable regularly. For instance, if homeopaths publish papers that suggest their remedies—which are bare of any active substance—cure cancer.[25] Often, nonsensical research happens when untrained and naive enthusiasts decide to dabble a bit in science in order to promote their trade. Here is a particularly striking example by Indian homeopaths[26]:

In the current scenario of medical sciences, homeopathy, the most popular system of therapy, is recognized as one of the components of complementary and alternative medicine (CAM) across the world. Despite, a long debate is continuing whether homeopathy is just a placebo or more than it, homeopathy has been considered to be safe and cost-effectiveness therapeutic modality. A number of human ailments ranging from common to serious have been treated with homeopathy. However, selection of appropriate medicines against a disease is cumbersome task as total spectrum of symptoms of a patient guides this process. Available data suggest that homeopathy has potency not only to treat various types of cancers but also to reduce the side effects caused by standard therapeutic modalities like chemotherapy, radiotherapy or surgery. Although homeopathy has been widely used for management of cancers, its efficacy is still under question. In the present review, the anti-cancer effect of various homeopathic drugs against different kinds of cancers has been discussed and future course of action has also been suggested.

[24] https://www.amazon.co.uk/More-Harm-than-Good-Complementary-ebook/dp/B078ZQXQNP/.

[25] Rostock M, Naumann J, Guethlin C, Guenther L, Bartsch HH, Walach H. Classical homeopathy in the treatment of cancer patients–a prospective observational study of two independent cohorts. BMC Cancer. 2011;11:19. Published 2011 Jan 17. https://doi.org/10.1186/1471-2407-11-19

[26] Yadav R, Jee B, Rao KS. How homeopathic medicine works in cancer treatment: deep insight from clinical to experimental studies. J Exp Ther Oncol. 2019 Jan;13(1):71–76. PMID: 30658031.

On other occasions, the authors of nonsensical research seem not naïve at all but know only too well what they are doing. Take for instance the plethora of 'pragmatic' trials which are designed such that their results must inevitably produce the positive result which the researchers intended to show.[27] Here researchers use a poor imitation of science for the purpose of promoting their business.

Nonsensical research is not merely a waste of resources, it is an unethical attempt to generate findings that mislead us all. Moreover, it gives science a bad name and can lead to patients' unwillingness to take part in necessary research. The damage done by nonsensical research projects is therefore immeasurable.

First Do no Harm

The sentence 'first do no harm' originates from the Hippocratic Oath which all doctors take when finishing medical school. Even though many people believe this to be true, it is not:

- Most doctors were never asked to take this oath.
- 'First do no harm' does not appear in the famous oath.

But doctors are surely obliged to 'first do no harm', because it is an important principle of medical ethics. This too is not entirely true, I am afraid. If it were, many doctors would have to stop practising. This is because clinicians cause harm all the time. As any cancer patient will know only too well, their injections hurt, their diagnostic procedures can be unpleasant and painful, their treatments cause significant adverse effects, their surgical interventions are full of risks, etc., etc.

Therefore, the ethical imperative of 'first do no harm' had to change. The current successor to the Hippocratic Oath, the Declaration of Geneva, was adopted by the World Medical Association (WMA) at its second General Assembly in 1948 affirming the ethical principles of the medical profession. The current version of the Declaration was adopted by the WMA General Assembly on 14 October 2017 and addresses key ethical issues[28]:

---

[27] Ernst E, Lee MS. A trial design that generates only "positive" results. *J Postgrad Med*. 2008;54(3):214–216. https://doi.org/10.4103/0022-3859.41806

[28] Parsa-Parsi RW. The Revised Declaration of Geneva: A Modern-Day Physician's Pledge. JAMA. 2017 Nov 28;318(20):1971–1972. https://doi.org/10.1001/jama.2017.16230. PMID: 29,049,507.

AS A MEMBER OF THE MEDICAL PROFESSION:

I SOLEMNLY PLEDGE to dedicate my life to the service of humanity;

THE HEALTH AND WELL-BEING OF MY PATIENT will be my first consideration;

I WILL RESPECT the autonomy and dignity of my patient;

I WILL MAINTAIN the utmost respect for human life;

I WILL NOT PERMIT considerations of age, disease or disability, creed, ethnic origin, gender, nationality, political affiliation, race, sexual orientation, social standing, or any other factor to intervene between my duty and my patient;

I WILL RESPECT the secrets that are confided in me, even after the patient has died;

I WILL PRACTISE my profession with conscience and dignity and in accordance with good medical practice;

I WILL FOSTER the honour and noble traditions of the medical profession;

I WILL GIVE to my teachers, colleagues, and students the respect and gratitude that is their due;

I WILL SHARE my medical knowledge for the benefit of the patient and the advancement of healthcare;

I WILL ATTEND TO my own health, well-being, and abilities in order to provide care of the highest standard;

I WILL NOT USE my medical knowledge to violate human rights and civil liberties, even under threat;

I MAKE THESE PROMISES solemnly, freely, and upon my honour.

Of course, healthcare professionals must be allowed to do even quite serious harm—as long as they have the health and the well-being of their patients as their first consideration. Thus, there is one essential precondition: their actions must be expected to generate more good than harm. This is particularly true for cancer care:

- If the known risks of a cancer treatment are greater than the expected benefits, it cannot ethically be prescribed.
- If the benefits of a cancer treatment outweigh the risks, we can consider it as a reasonable therapeutic option, even if its potential for harm is considerable.

But this can, of course, be applied to treatments where both the risks and the benefits are well-understood. What about the many SCAMs where there is uncertainty regarding one or both of these factors? This question is impossible to answer in the abstract. Clinicians need to look at the best evidence for each specific case (see Sects. 1.2, 1.3 and 1.4 of this book) and must, together with the patient, try to arrive at an informed decision.

Informed Consent

Informed consent is a basic ethical principle and a precondition for any therapeutic intervention or diagnostic test, regardless of whether it is administered in research or clinical practice. Essentially, there are four elements to informed consent:

1. the patient must have decision-making capacity,
2. the patient's decision must be free from coercion or manipulation,
3. all relevant information must be disclosed to the patient,
4. patients must understand what they have been told.

There is general agreement that 'all relevant information' should include the following points:

- the nature of the condition to be treated,
- the nature of the procedure,
- the evidence regarding its effectiveness,
- the evidence about risks,
- other treatments that might be used, including the option of doing nothing at all.

If we carefully consider these 5 points, we soon realise that, in terms of informed consent, there are profound differences between SCAM and conventional medicine. These differences relate not so much to the nature of the procedures but more crucially to the competence of the practitioners.

At medical school, students learn the necessary facts that should enable them to adequately deal with the information listed above. (This does not necessarily mean that, in conventional medical or surgical practice, informed consent is always optimal; yet there is little doubt that, in theory, it can be adequate.) By contrast, SCAM practitioners have not normally been to medical school. They will have gone through an entirely different type of training, sometimes even through none at all. Therefore, the question arises whether—even in theory—they would be able to relate to their patients all the above-listed information necessary for informed consent.

Addressing this question by looking at concrete cases might make this situation clearer. Consider the case of a patient suffering from frequent headaches (which will later turn out to be caused by a malignant brain tumour) who consults four different SCAM practitioners:

- an acupuncturist,
- a homeopath,
- a naturopath,
- a traditional herbalist.

The question is, are these practitioners able to convey all the relevant information to their patient before starting their treatments?

THE TRADITIONAL ACUPUNCTURIST

- Can he provide full information about the condition? The patient might be treated for an assumed 'energy blockage'; other diagnoses might not be given adequate consideration.
- Can he explain the nature of the procedure? Yes.
- Can he explain its potential benefits? He is likely to have an over-optimistic view on this issue.
- Can he explain its risks? Perhaps.
- Can he provide details about the other options, including the option of doing nothing at all? No.

THE CLASSICAL HOMEOPATH

- Can he provide full information about the condition? No, a classical homeopath considers the totality of the symptoms to be the valid diagnosis.
- Can he explain the nature of the procedure? Yes.
- Can he explain its potential benefits? Doubtful.
- Can he explain its risks? Doubtful.
- Can he provide details about the other options, including the option of doing nothing at all? No.

THE NATUROPATH

- Can he provide full information about the condition? Doubtful.
- Can he explain the nature of the procedure? Yes.

- Can he explain its potential benefits? He is likely to have an over-optimistic view on this.
- Can he explain its risks? Doubtful.
- Can he provide details about the other options, including the option of doing nothing at all? No.

THE TRADITIONAL HERBALIST

- Can he provide full information about the condition? No.
- Can he explain the nature of the procedure? Yes.
- Can he explain its potential benefits? He is likely to have an over-optimistic view on this.
- Can he explain its risks? He is likely to have a too optimistic view on this.
- Can he provide details about the other options, including the option of doing nothing at all? No.

The answers provided to the above questions are based on my experience of more than 25 years with SCAM practitioners in the UK, Germany and Austria; I am aware of the degree of simplification required to give short, succinct replies. The answers are, of course, assumptions as well as generalisations. There may well be individual practitioners who would do better (or worse) than the fictitious average I had in mind when answering the questions. Moreover, one would expect important national differences.

My answers nevertheless suggest that, in SCAM, as provided by non-medically trained practitioners, fully informed consent is rarely, if ever, possible. If that is so, SCAM practitioners regularly violate the rules of medical ethics. Or, to put it bluntly: the ethical practice of SCAM is rarely possible.

1.7   What Is Reliable Evidence?

Some people engage in seemingly endless discussions around the nature and importance of evidence. Many SCAM enthusiasts claim, for instance, that their experience is at least as important as scientific evidence. Others say that SCAM cannot be squeezed into the straightjacket of scientific testing and that evidence is thus irrelevant. But are such arguments valid?

In this chapter, I will try to analyse some of the issues related to evidence as they apply to SCAM and cancer. In doing so, I will abstain from naming any specific form of SCAM. This discussion should not be about the value of this or that particular SCAM; it is about more fundamental issues which often get confused.

Clinical Experience Is Notoriously Unreliable

Whenever their patients get better, clinicians invariably assume this to be the result of their treatments. Naturally, patients feel much the same. Both might, however, be mistaken. Two events, the treatment and the improvement, that follow each other in time are not necessarily causally related. Correlation is not causation! We all know that, of course. So, we ought to consider alternative explanations for a patient's improvement after receiving a therapy.

Let's use the example of a cancer patient suffering from fatigue who uses a SCAM and subsequently feels better. There are several reasons why she might have improved, even if the SCAM was ineffective, i.e. not better than a placebo:

- Fatigue often wears off over time, even if we do nothing at all (natural history of the condition).
- If we quantify any symptom repeatedly while it is at its peak, it is statistically likely to be less severe the second time round (regression towards the mean).
- The expectation of getting better will contribute to the patient's improvement (placebo effect).
- Patients often use concomitant treatments in parallel, in which case it is difficult to say which therapy caused the positive outcome.

These and other phenomena can contribute to the clinical outcome in such a way that ineffective treatments appear to be effective. What follows is plausible for scientists, yet counter-intuitive for clinicians and their patients: the prescribed treatment is only one of many factors that determine the clinical outcome. And because of this, even the most impressive clinical experience of the perceived effectiveness of a treatment can be totally misleading.

Enthusiasts of SCAM find all this hard to believe and often have counter-arguments, for instance:

1. The improvement was so prompt that it was evidently caused by the SCAM [this notion is unconvincing; placebo effects can be just as immediate].

2. I have seen it happen so many times that it cannot be a coincidence [some practitioners are very caring, charismatic, or empathetic; they will thus regularly generate powerful placebo-responses].
3. A study with several thousand patients shows that 75% of them improved with my SCAM [such response rates are not uncommon, even for ineffective treatments, if patient-expectation was high].
4. Chronic conditions don't suddenly get better by themselves; my SCAM can therefore not be a placebo [this is incorrect, eventually many chronic conditions improve, if only temporarily].
5. I had a patient with cancer, who received my treatment and was cured [if one investigates such cases, one often finds that the patient also used conventional treatments. Moreover, in rare instances, even cancer patients experience spontaneous remissions].
6. I have tried the SCAM myself and had a positive outcome [nobody is immune to the multifactorial nature of the perceived clinical response].
7. Even children and animals respond very well to my SCAM, surely they are not prone to placebo effects [animals can be conditioned to respond; and then there are, of course, the natural history of the disease, and the placebo effect by proxy].

This is not to say that clinical experience is useless. I am merely pointing out that, when it comes to determining the effectiveness of the therapy, clinical experience is no substitute for evidence. Experience is invaluable for a lot of other reasons, but it can at best be an indicator and never a proof of the effectiveness of a therapy.

What then Is Reliable Evidence?

As the clinical outcomes after treatments always have many determinants, we need a different approach, if we want to know whether the therapy itself was helpful. Essentially, we need to know what would have happened if our patients had not received the SCAM in question.

The above-outlined multifactorial nature of any clinical response requires controlling for all the factors that might determine the outcome other than the treatment per se. Ideally, we would need to create a situation where two groups of patients are exposed to the full range of factors, while the only difference is that one group does receive the treatment, while the other one does not. Bingo! This is precisely the principle of a controlled clinical trial (Fig. 1.1).

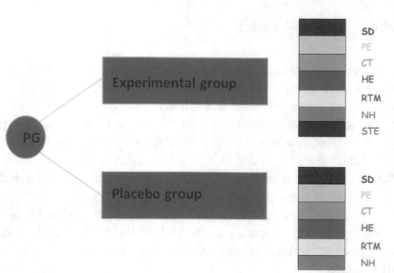

Fig. 1.1 Schematic drawing of the factors determining the outcome of a clinical trial: A patient group (PG) is divided into two sub-groups, the experimental and the control group; they are exposed to the same influences except for the specific therapeutic effect (STE) of the treatment that is being tested. Thus, any difference in outcomes will be due to the STE. NH = natural history of the disease, RMT = regression towards the mean, HE = Hathorne effect, CT = concomitant treatments, PE = placebo effect, SD = social desirability [copyright E Ernst]

Such studies are designed to minimise all possible sources of bias and confounding. By definition, they have a control group which means that, at the end of the treatment period, we can compare the effects of the treatment in question with those of:

- another intervention,
- a placebo,
- or no treatment at all.

Many different variations of the controlled trial exist so that the experiment can be adapted to the requirements of the particular treatment and the specific research question at hand. The overriding principle, however, is always the same: we want to make sure that we can reliably determine whether the treatment (and not some other co-determinant of the outcome) was the true cause of the clinical effect.

Reliability of Clinical Trials

Unfortunately, not all clinical trials produce reliable results. There are many ways in which investigators might mislead us with seemingly sound studies.

Pilot studies are small scale preliminary trials for evaluating feasibility, time, cost, adverse events, and improve upon the study design prior to performance of a full-scale research project. Yet, the elementary preconditions are not fulfilled by the plethora of SCAM pilot studies that are currently being published. True pilot studies of SCAM are, in fact, very rare. The danger of this abundance of pseudo-pilots is obvious: they can easily be interpreted as showing encouragingly positive results for whatever SCAM is being tested. Subsequently, SCAM proponents can mislead the public by claiming that there are plenty of positive studies and therefore their SCAM is supported by sound evidence.

Researchers of SCAM often employ study designs that can only generate positive findings. The most popular one is the 'A + B versus B' design. In a recent study, for instance, cancer patients suffering from fatigue were randomised to receive usual care or usual care plus regular acupuncture.[29] The researchers then monitored the patients' experience of fatigue and found that the acupuncture group did significantly better than the control group. Thus acupuncture appeared to be effective which might well be a false-negative conclusion. Imagine you have an amount of money A and your friend owns the same sum plus another amount B. Who has more money? It is, of course, your friend: A + B will always be more than A [unless B is a negative amount]. For the same reason, trials with an 'A + B versus B' design will always generate positive results [unless the treatment in question does actual harm]. Routine care plus acupuncture is more than routine care alone, and the former is, therefore, more than likely to produce a better result, even if acupuncture is a pure placebo—after all, a placebo is more than nothing, and the placebo effect will impact on the outcome, particularly if we are dealing with a highly subjective symptom such as fatigue.

Another method that generates false-positive results is to omit blinding. The purpose of blinding the patient, the therapist and the evaluator of the outcomes in clinical trials are to make sure that expectation is not a contributor to the outcome. Expectation might not move mountains, but it can

[29] Molassiotis A, Bardy J, Finnegan-John J, Mackereth P, Ryder DW, Filshie J, Ream E, Richardson A. Acupuncture for cancer-related fatigue in patients with breast cancer: a pragmatic randomized controlled trial. J Clin Oncol. 2012 Dec 20;30(36):4470–6. https://doi.org/10.1200/JCO.2012.41.6222. Ep 2012 Oct 29. PMID: 23109700.

certainly influence the result of a clinical trial.[30] Patients who have reason to hope getting better because they receive therapy regularly do get better, even if that therapy is entirely useless.

Failure to randomise is another source of bias which can mislead us.[31] If we allow patients or trialists to select or chose which patients receive the experimental and which get the control treatment, it is likely that the two groups differ in a number of variables. Some of these variables might, in turn, impact on the outcome. If, for instance, doctors allocate their patients to the experimental and control groups, they might select those who will respond to the former and those who don't to the latter. This may not happen intentionally but through intuition or instinct: responsible health care professionals want those patients who have the most need to benefit from a given treatment to receive that treatment. Only randomisation can, when done properly, make sure we are comparing comparable groups of patients, and non-randomisation is likely to produce misleading findings.

Some studies do not test whether an experimental treatment is superior to another one (often called superiority trials), but assess whether it is equivalent to a therapy that is generally accepted to be effective. The idea is that, if both treatments produce similarly positive results, they must be both effective. For instance, such a study might compare the effects of acupuncture to a common pain-killer. Such trials are called non-superiority or equivalence trials, and they offer a wide range of possibilities for misleading us. If, for example, such a trial has not enough patients, it might show no difference where, in fact, there is one.

Another way in which clinical trials can mislead us is to administer a treatment to the control group that is either under-dosed, wrongly timed, not indicated or harmful. The trick here is to make sure that the intervention in the control group cannot generate a positive result. In such scenarios, even the most useless SCAM would appear to be effective simply because it is more effective or less harmful than the comparator.

A variation of this theme is the plethora of controlled clinical trials comparing one unproven therapy to another unproven treatment. The results are likely to indicate that there is no difference in the clinical outcome experienced by the patients in the two groups. Enthusiastic SCAM researchers then

[30] Atlas LY, Whittington RA, Lindquist MA, Wielgosz J, Sonty N, Wager TD. Dissociable influences of opiates and expectations on pain. J Neurosci. 2012 Jun 6;32(23):8053–64. https://doi.org/10.1523/JNEUROSCI.0383-12.2012. PMID: 22674280; PMCID: PMC3387557.

[31] Odgaard-Jensen J, Vist GE, Timmer A, Kunz R, Akl EA, Schünemann H, Briel M, Nordmann AJ, Pregno S, Oxman AD. Randomisation to protect against selection bias in healthcare trials. Cochrane Database Syst Rev. 2011 Apr 13;2011(4):MR000012. https://doi.org/10.1002/14651858.MR000012.pub3. PMID: 21,491,415; PMCID: PMC7150228.

tend to conclude that this proves both treatments to be equally effective. The truth, however, may well be that both treatments were similarly useless.

Systematic Reviews

So, clinical trials are not necessarily perfect. They can have many flaws and have often been criticised for their inherent limitations. It is therefore wise not to rely on the findings of a single study. Independent replications are usually required before we can be reasonably sure. Unfortunately, the findings of such replications do not always confirm the results of the previous study. Consequently, we may end up with a confusing mixture of positive and negative findings. Whenever that happens, it is tempting to cherry-pick those studies which seem to confirm our prior belief – tempting perhaps, but certainly wrong. In order to arrive at the most reliable conclusion about the effectiveness of any treatment, we must consider the totality of the reliable evidence. This goal is best achieved by conducting what experts call a 'systematic review'.

In a systematic review, we assess the quality and quantity of the totality of the available evidence, try to synthesise the findings and arrive at an overall verdict about the treatment in question. Technically speaking, this process minimises selection and random biases. Systematic reviews and meta-analyses (these are systematic reviews that pool the data of individual studies and thus arrive at a new quantitative result) therefore constitute, according to a broad consensus, the best available evidence for or against the effectiveness of any treatment. In the following sections of this book, I rely where possible on such evidence when discussing the effectiveness of SCAM.

Why Is Evidence Important?

In a way, this question has already been answered: only with reliable evidence can we tell with any degree of certainty that it was the treatment per se—and not any of the other factors mentioned above—that caused any clinical effect. Only if we have such evidence can we be certain about cause and effect. And only then can we make sure that cancer patients receive the best possible treatments currently available.

There are, of course, those in SCAM who claim that causality does not matter all that much. What is paramount, they say, is to help the patient. Even if it was a placebo effect that reduced the cancer-related fatigue, who cares? What is important is that the patient got rid of her symptoms.

This sounds compassionate, but there are many reasons why this attitude is nevertheless misguided. To mention just one: we all might agree that the placebo effect can benefit many patients, yet it would be wrong to assume that we need a placebo treatment to generate a placebo-response. If a clinician administers an effective therapy [one that generates benefit beyond placebo] with compassion, time, empathy and understanding, she will generate a placebo-response PLUS a response to the therapy administered. In this case, the patient benefits twice. It follows that merely administering a placebo is less than optimal; in fact, it usually means preventing the patient from benefiting from an effective therapy.

We probably can all agree that helping the patient is the most important task of a clinician. This task is best achieved by maximising the non-specific [e.g. placebo] effects, while making sure that the patient benefits from the specific effects of what evidence-based medicine has to offer. That is our goal in good clinical practice, and therefore we need both reliable evidence and experience. One cannot be a substitute for the other, and scientific evidence is an essential precondition for good medicine. Chaps. 2, 3 and 4 will focus on outlining the evidence for and against SCAM for cancer.

1.8 Pseudoscience and Pseudoscientists

Pseudoscience is defined as a system of theories or assertions about the natural world that claim or appear to be scientific but that, in fact, are not. In a way, pseudoscience is a caricature of science—a caricature, I hasten to add, that is not funny but dangerous. And because it is dangerous, it would be helpful, if cancer victims and their carers were able to tell it from real science.

However, the demarcation of pseudoscience and science is far from straightforward and remains an unsolved issue. Popper's principle that to be scientific, a hypothesis must be falsifiable is probably correct, but of little practical use for cancer patients wanting to protect themselves from pseudoscience and pseudoscientists.

Pseudoscientists seem to love SCAM, and proponents of SCAM love pseudoscience. To shield us from the dangers of pseudoscience, it might be helpful to analyse the methods and techniques pseudoscientists regularly employ for fooling us (and often also themselves). Here is a list that could be useful.

1. Pseudoscientists ignore settled issues in science: A simple example is the claim of many SCAM providers that cancer is caused by a psychological trauma or conflict (for instance, New German Medicine, Sect. 3.5). We

long know that the assumption is false, yet it lives on in many forms of SCAM. Pseudoscience is often akin to science denial.[32]

2. They aim to further their business, ideology etc.: The aim of science is to generate objective, valid and reliable knowledge. This aim is not shared by pseudoscientists who often conduct research to advance their own interests. e.g.[33] While scientists want to create progress, pseudoscientists create regress.

3. They misapply real science: Quantum mechanics is of little practical use in healthcare. Yet, pseudoscientists ignore this fact and claim that quantum mechanics explains the actions of their SCAMs.[34] As few people understand quantum mechanics (including the SCAM providers who make the claim) this would impress some consumers. In any case, quantum babble always looks 'cutting edge' and is good for business.

4. They reject scientific standards: Science has established standards of evidence and experiment to ensure that data generated through science are reliable. Pseudoscientists are either ignorant of these standards, disregard them, or even denounce them as an obsolete paradigm that does not apply to their endeavours.

5. They deny that any hypotheses worth the name must be falsifiable: Pseudoscientists frequently make claims which cannot be shown to be wrong. Consequently, they claim that they are correct. For instance, the life force assumed in various forms of SCAM to be responsible for our health cannot easily be shown not to exist. Science is not a good tool for demonstrating the absence of a phenomenon. Therefore, proponents of SCAM feel that their assumptions must be correct.

6. They rely on anecdotes instead of evidence. Pseudoscientists tend to ignore the fact that anecdotes tell us little about cause and effect (Sect. 1.7). The reason for this preference is obvious: there are plenty of anecdotes seemingly supporting SCAM, while sound evidence is scarce and often not in SCAM's favour.

7. They use words in an incorrect or misleading manner: For example, energy, meridians, quantum effects, subluxations, as used in SCAM, are terms that have a different meaning than in science.

---

[32] Hansson SO. Science denial as a form of pseudoscience. Stud Hist Philos Sci. 2017 Jun;63:39–47. https://doi.org/10.1016/j.shpsa.2017.05.002. Epub 2017 May 31. PMID: 28629651.

[33] Beuth J, Schneider B, VAN Leendert R, Uhlenbruck G. Large-scale Survey of the Impact of Complementary Medicine on Side-effects of Adjuvant Hormone Therapy in Patients with Breast Cancer. In Vivo. 2016 Jan-Feb;30(1):73–5. PMID: 26709132.

[34] Ross CL. Energy Medicine: Current Status and Future Perspectives. Glob Adv Health Med. 2019 Feb 27;8:2,164,956,119,831,221. https://doi.org/10.1177/2164956119831221. PMID: 30834177; PMCID: PMC6396053.

8. They employ pseudoscientific language: Clarity of language is an essential element for effective communication in science. Using the example of bioresonance therapy, one can demonstrate how pseudoscientific language is employed not to clarify but to cloud important issues. Such attempts to present nonsense as science mislead patients and can thus endanger their health.[35]

9. They employ logical fallacies: Fallacious arguments used by pseudoscientists have been discussed in Sect. 1.4. They include, for instance, the appeal to authority or the appeal to tradition. Fallacies often convince unsuspecting cancer patients, yet they are misleading and deceptive notions.

10. They claim to be suppressed: Whenever pseudoscience is rejected by science because it does not conform to accepted standards, pseudoscientists claim to be suppressed, and the scientific community is depicted as a dangerous hegemony that rejects new ideas in order to perpetuate their grip on power. Conspiracy theories which posit that 'the establishment' is determined to suppress the views or findings of SCAM proponents (Chap. 6).

11. They draw conclusions not supported by the evidence: Pseudoscientists conduct studies not to test their assumptions, their aim is to support a preordained conclusion. Thus, they often engage in excessive logical leaps when the data is insufficient to support the desired conclusion. e.g.[36] This often goes as far as enabling them to draw a positive conclusion on the basis of negative data.

12. They misrepresent the evidence: Pseudoscientists often argue that their approaches are supported by a select number of publications from important organisations. However, upon reading such literature it becomes apparent that the articles supplied do not report what was claimed and that there is no or very little empirical or theoretical support for the claim.

13. They cherry-pick their evidence: Pseudoscientists regularly offer evidence in support of their SCAM, while omitting the fact that there are many more studies that contradict their claim. Scientists, by contrast, present the totality of all reliable evidence (Sect. 1.7).

14. They focus on the fringes: Science regularly generates anomalous data and anecdotal findings that are inconsistent with the wider consensus.

---

[35] Ernst E. Bioresonance, a study of pseudo-scientific language. Forsch Komplementarmed Klass Naturheilkd. 2004 Jun;11(3):171–3. https://doi.org/10.1159/000079446. PMID: 15249751.

[36] Acupressure: when all else fails, ignore the results and publish a favourable conclusion (edzardernst.com).

Pseudoscientists present such anomalies as a coherent body of knowledge that supports the overthrow of existing knowledge.

15. They doubt the competence of scientists: For example, if an academic raises concerns about a particular SCAM, pseudoscientists might point out that, without having attended courses and seminars, the academic does not have the required understanding and his criticism is of no value. Thus only an experienced homeopath is competent to issue acceptable criticism of homeopathy, for instance. As any experienced homeopath is by definition a convinced homeopath, acceptable criticism is non-existent.

16. They claim that science is not yet advanced enough to explain their SCAM: When criticised, pseudoscientists suggest that they are attacked because their revolutionary approach is ahead of its time. Often they refer to a quote attributed to Arthur Schopenhauer: 'All truth passes through three stages. First, it is ridiculed. Second, it is violently opposed. Third, it is accepted as self-evident'. As Carl Sagan pointed out, the fact that some geniuses were laughed at does not imply that all who are laughed at are geniuses. They laughed at Columbus, they laughed at Fulton, they laughed at the Wright brothers. But they also laughed at Bozo the Clown.

17. They fail to connect to other relevant areas of research: For example, homeopaths assume that homeopathic remedies become stronger as they get more diluted, and that water has memory. Both of these claims run counter to established scientific knowledge from physics and chemistry (Sect. 3.2).

18. They avoid self-correction: Self-correction is an essential and powerful mechanism by which science eliminates errors. Pseudoscientists hardly ever learn from mistakes, instead they perpetuate errors even in the face of overwhelming evidence.

19. They abuse peer-review: Scientific papers must be peer-reviewed, i.e. checked and criticised by independent experts, before they get published. Pseudoscientists have created SCAM journals where this process is abused by allowing researchers who share their pseudoscientific views to do the checking. Thus any critical input is by-passed and peer-review is degraded to a mere farce.[37]

20. They are consumed with evangelic zeal and issue legal threats or ad hominem attacks: Pseudoscientists find it impossible to accept or

---

[37] Some alternative medicine journals should be de-listed (edzardernst.com).

consider well-reasoned criticism. When they run out of arguments, pseudoscientists regularly attack their opponents verbally or try to issue libel actions against them.[38] The aim, of course, is to silence the critic.

I listed these 20 activities in the hope that cancer patients and their carers might find them helpful for identifying pseudoscientists and averting the harm they can do. Essentially, they are characteristic of a person who is dishonest and aims at misleading us about SCAM. It seems self-evident that such a person can seduce cancer patients to make therapeutic choices that are sub-optimal or even harmful.

But please, don't get me wrong: none of these characteristics on their own is enough to tell with any degree of security a pseudoscientist from a scientist. Cherry-picking evidence, evangelic zeal, ad hominem attacks, etc. are all phenomena that sadly occur also outside pseudoscience. I, therefore, suggest to consider the totality of the items on my list. The more of them are met in any specific case, the more likely it is that we are dealing with a pseudoscientist.

1.9   How to Best Use the Following Sections of This Book

The next sections of this book are dedicated to the evidence for or against SCAM as it pertains to

- Cancer prevention (Chap. 2)
- Cancer cures (Chap. 3)
- Supportive and palliative cancer care (Chap. 4)

As I wanted them to be as evidence-based as possible, I needed to supply references to the most relevant research articles. Where possible, I quoted up-to-date systematic reviews (Sect. 1.8) by independent authorities or myself. To make things as clear as possible, I concluded the discussion of each specific SCAM with this standard table.

Plausibility
Effectiveness
Safety

(continued)

---

[38] Bonneux L. The Singh libel case and 'alternative medicine'. Eur J Public Health. 2009 Dec;19(6):574–5. https://doi.org/10.1093/eurpub/ckp175. Epub 2009 Nov 2. PMID: 19884159.

(continued)

Cost
Risk/benefit balance

The five criteria used in these tables require some explanations:

- PLAUSIBILITY addresses the question of whether the basic assumptions on which the SCAM is based are in line with the laws of nature and our current medical knowledge. For instance, the notion of reflexologists that specific areas on the soles of our feet correspond to specific organ systems is implausible, because it contradicts the basic facts from anatomy and physiology. By contrast, the claim that a herbal remedy is effective is plausible, because plants contain chemicals that might have pharmacological activity.
- EFFECTIVENESS deals with the question whether according to the best available evidence, a SCAM works. My specific question usually is, does it work better than a placebo? When evaluating the evidence, it is, of course, important to also consider the quality of the published studies.
- SAFETY addresses the question of whether the SCAM per se can do harm. Here, I usually omit all indirect risks of SCAM. Yet, such indirect risks can be significant, for instance, if a SCAM is promoted as an alternative cure for cancer.
- COST provides a rough judgement on the expense associated with the SCAM. Here I also considered whether a therapy usually requires more than one session which would, of course, increase the total expense.
- RISK/BENEFIT BALANCE combines the issues of effectiveness and safety by asking whether the SCAM in question generates more good than harm. Here, it is crucial to remember two things. Firstly, the risk/benefit balance cannot be positive, even for a totally harmless SCAM, if it has not been documented to be effective. Secondly, it is wise for cancer patients to only employ treatments that do more good than harm.

With these tables, I attempt to offer my assessments by using just three very simple grades:

- positive
- debatable
- negative
- in a few cases, I found it impossible to decide and used two grades simultaneously to indicate that the truth lies somewhere in between.

On the one hand, such simplicity is desirable for accessibility and easy reading. On the other hand, it does not allow much subtlety and nuance. When making these judgement calls, I often had to rely on more evidence than I was able to cite in the text. Therefore, they represent my overall assessments based on the collective evidence from many years of research.

The tables are meant to complement the text; together they give you a quick and reliable idea whether the SCAM in question might be of value for you. My evaluations are deliberately critical. As cancer patients are already exposed to an abundance of uncritical promotion of useless and even dangerous SCAMs, this approach is the best way to assist you in finding your way through the disorientating maze of misinformation that often characterises SCAM.

2

Prevention

Prevention is the act of stopping something from happening. In healthcare, it entails measures that stop disease from occurring. Many proponents of SCAM are convinced that SCAM has an important role to play in cancer prevention. This is easily demonstrated by even just glancing at the many books on the subject. Two examples must suffice:

1. *Most cancer research dollars have been wasted by asking the wrong questions, looking in the wrong places, and recycling the same failed approaches while expecting different results. Conventional cancer treatments damage health, cause new cancers, lower the quality of life, and decrease the chances of survival. In fact, most people who die from cancer are not dying from cancer, but from their treatments! That's the bad news. Here's the good news: We can end the cancer epidemic. In Never Fear Cancer Again, readers will gain a revolutionary new understanding of health and disease and will come to understand that cancer is a biological process that can be turned on and off, not something that can be surgically removed or destroyed with radiation or toxic chemicals. So whether cancer has already been diagnosed or if prevention is the concern, it is possible to turn off the wayward production of these malfunctioning cells once and for all by reading this book and implementing its strategies. The key to any disease has one simple cause: malfunctioning cells that are created by either deficiency or toxicity. By switching off the malfunctioning cells, you switch off cancer. Never Fear Cancer Again guides readers*

E. Ernst, *So-Called Alternative Medicine (SCAM) for Cancer*, https://doi.org/10.1007/978-3-030-74158-7_2

along six pathways that cause deficiency or toxicity at the cellular level: nutritional path, genetic path, medical path, toxin path, physical path, and the psychological path. By making key lifestyle changes, people truly have the power to take control of cancer and transform their health. This radically different, yet holistic approach restored author Raymond Francis back to health just as it has helped thousands of others, many of whom were told they had no other options or that their cancer was incurable. Take back your health with this book and never fear cancer again.[1]

2. *The immune system is the primary defense mechanism of our body to fight cancer. Cancer cells and pathogens can spread quickly in the body, when the immune system is weak. Only an intact immune system manages to eliminate the hostile cells. Strengthening the immune system therefore is extremely important for the prevention of cancer. In this homeopathic and naturopathic adviser, I will give you recommendations on how to prevent cancer with Homeopathy, Schuessler salts (also named cell salts, tissue salts) and herbal tinctures. I will present you with the most-proven homeopathic remedies and Schuessler salts, including the appropriate potency and dosage. I wish you much success, joy of life and especially your health.*[2]

Equally disturbing are the many conferences misinforming laypeople about SCAM and cancer prevention. Here is an announcement from a UK charity:

> … the weekends feature a breathtaking line-up of over 40 expert speakers. On this first weekend, … the event focuses on an Introduction to Integrative Medicine, with speakers covering topics including lifestyle changes, supplements and the role of the microbiome in cancer care and prevention.[3]

Yes, prevention is undoubtedly better than cure. The decline in cancer mortality is owed to a large extent to the success of implementing preventative measures. But how effective is SCAM in preventing cancers? Between 30 and 50% of all cancer cases are said to be preventable. So, the potential could be enormous. Conventional cancer prevention strategies focus mainly on the elimination or reduction of the following risk factors:

- Tobacco, the single greatest avoidable risk factor for cancer mortality (Fig. 2.1)

---

[1] https://www.amazon.co.uk/Never-Fear-Cancer-Again-Revolutionary/dp/075731550X/.

[2] https://www.amazon.co.uk/Cancer-Prevention-Homeopathy-Schuessler-homeopathic-ebook/dp/B07 DR1K5HZ/.

[3] https://yestolife.org.uk/event/your-life-and-cancer-2020-1/.

- Physical inactivity
- Dietary factors
- Obesity and being overweight
- Alcohol
- Infections, approximately 15% of all cancers are attributable to infectious agents such as helicobacter pylori, human papilloma virus (HPV), hepatitis B and C, and Epstein-Barr virus.
- Environmental pollution
- Occupational carcinogens
- Radiation.

These strategies are undoubtedly effective. For instance, the Mediterranean diet, the intake of vegetables, wholegrains, fish, poultry, coffee, macronutrients such as monounsaturated fats and micronutrients are associated with a reduced risk of hepatocellular carcinoma.[4] Similarly, cooking habits, diet, passive smoking are related to lung cancer in non-smoking women.[5] And the decline of smoking during the last decades was by far the most influential factor in the fight against lung cancer.[6] To achieve these goals, an epic effort had been necessary in terms of research (currently, Medline lists >360,000 articles on the subject of cancer prevention), lobbying, politics, legal actions, etc. In it, SCAM played virtually no role at all.

None of the preventative approaches listed above belongs to the realm of SCAM (even though some SCAM-proponents seem to pretend otherwise), and we may well ask what precisely is the contribution of SCAM in cancer prevention?

If we search for SCAMs that demonstrably lower the risk of specific cancers, we are bound to get disappointed. Even ardent SCAM-proponents cannot but admit this fact:

Although there are no proven methods to definitively prevent cancer in either conventional medicine or cancer complementary and alternative medicine (CAM), many cancer prevention approaches currently under investigation

---

[4] George ES, Sood S, Broughton A, Cogan G, Hickey M, Chan WS, Sudan S, Nicoll AJ. The Association between Diet and Hepatocellular Carcinoma: A Systematic Review. Nutrients. 2021 Jan 8;13(1):E172. http://doi.org/10.3390/nu13010172. PMID: 33430001.

[5] Huang J, Yue N, Shi N, Wang Q, Cui T, Ying H, Wang Z, Leng J, Sui Z, Xu Y, Wei B, Jin H. Influencing factors of lung cancer in nonsmoking women: systematic review and meta-analysis. J Public Health (Oxf). 2021 Jan 12:fdaa254. http://doi.org/10.1093/pubmed/fdaa254. Epub ahead of print. PMID: 33429425.

[6] Chang JT, Anic GM, Rostron BL, Tanwar M, Chang CM. Cigarette Smoking Reduction and Health Risks: A Systematic Review and Meta-Analysis. Nicotine Tob Res. 2020 Aug 17:ntaa156. http://doi.org/10.1093/ntr/ntaa156. Epub ahead of print. PMID: 32803250.

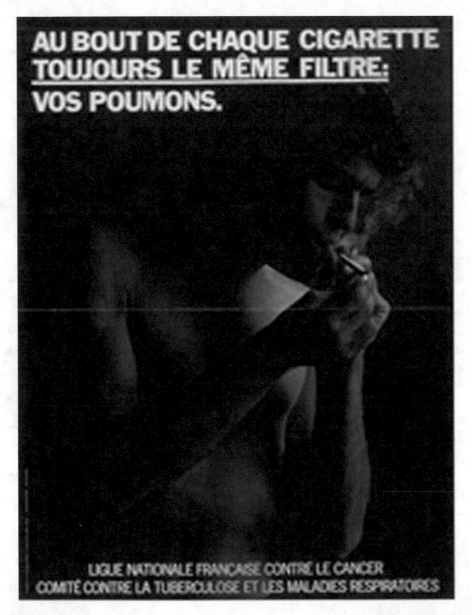

Fig. 2.1 French government warning about smoking, 'at the end of each cigarette, there is always the same filter; your lungs'. *Source* US National Library of Medicine

focus on dietary changes, nutritional supplements, lifestyle modifications (e.g., increasing exercise, decreasing sun exposure), and decreasing environmental exposures, many of which fall into the field of CAM research. Although the field of research on CAM in treatment of diseases, including cancer, has exploded in the past few years, there is a notable lag in the development of research protocols in the area of cancer prevention.[7]

In this chapter, I will summarise the existing evidence on the topic of SCAM as preventative measures for reducing the risks of acquiring cancer.

Flax

Flax (linseed, Linum usitatissimum) is a plant from in the *Linaceae* family which is cultivated for food, fibre (for making linen) and oil production. Flaxseed contains protein, dietary fibre, several B vitamins, and minerals. Dietary supplements containing flax have been associated with a range of positive effects on health. Flax is known for its lignan, α-linolenic acid, and fibre content, components that are claimed to possess phyto-oestrogenic, anti-inflammatory, and hormone modulating effects.

A systematic review evaluated the effects of flax consumption on the risk of breast cancer incidence or recurrence. The authors found only two randomised clinical trials (RCTs). They concluded that *current evidence suggests that flax may be associated with decreased risk of breast cancer. Flax demonstrates antiproliferative effects in breast tissue of women at risk of breast cancer and may protect against primary breast cancer. Mortality risk may also be reduced among those living with breast cancer.*[8] This means that there is some positive evidence; but at present, it is far from convincing.

Plausibility	👍
Effectiveness	👎

(continued)

---

[7] https://link.springer.com/chapter/10.1007%2F978-3-030-15935-1_9.

[8] Flower G, Fritz H, Balneaves LG, et al. Flax and Breast Cancer: A Systematic Review. *Integr Cancer Ther.* 2014;13(3):181–192. http://doi.org/10.1177/1534735413502076.

(continued)

Safety	👍
Cost	👍
Risk/benefit balance	👍

Garlic

Garlic (*Allium sativum*) has been used for cooking since ancient times. It also has many pharmacological activities, most of which are directed towards the cardiovascular system.[9] The anti-cancer activity of garlic may be ascribed to the organosulfur compounds that are found in crushed garlic preparations. These compounds have been shown to inhibit different stages of cancer.[10]

Based on epidemiological studies, associations between garlic intake and colon, prostate, oesophageal, larynx, oral, ovary, and renal cell cancers have been reported.[11] A protective effect of garlic on gastric cancer mortality has also been noted.[12] Further epidemiological data suggest that eating raw garlic at least twice per week is inversely associated with liver cancer.[13] Finally, several animal studies seem to suggest that garlic has anti-cancer activity.[14]

---

[9] Pittler MH, Ernst E. Clinical effectiveness of garlic (Allium sativum). Mol Nutr Food Res. 2007 Nov;51(11):1382–5. http://doi.org/10.1002/mnfr.200700073. PMID: 17918163.

[10] Kaschula CH, Tuveri R, Ngarande F., Dzobo K, Barnett C, Kusza DA, Graham LM, Katz AA, Rafudeen MS, Parker MI, Hunter R, Schäfer G. The garlic compound ajoene covalently binds vimentin, disrupts the vimentin network and exerts anti-metastatic activity in cancer cells. BMC Cancer. 2019 Mar 20;19(1):248. http://doi.org/10.1186/s12885-019-5388-8. PMID: 30894168; PMCID: PMC6425727.

[11] Ansary J, Forbes-Hernández TY, Gil E, et al. Potential Health Benefit of Garlic Based on Human Intervention Studies: A Brief Overview. *Antioxidants (Basel).* 2020;9(7):619. Published 2020 Jul 15. http://doi.org/10.3390/antiox9070619.

[12] Guo Y, Li ZX, Zhang JY, et al. Association Between Lifestyle Factors, Vitamin and Garlic Supplementation, and Gastric Cancer Outcomes: A Secondary Analysis of a Randomized Clinical Trial. *JAMA Netw Open.* 2020;3(6):e206628. Published 2020 Jun 1. http://doi.org/10.1001/jamanetworkopen.2020.6628.

[13] Liu X, Baecker A, Wu M, Zhou JY, Yang J, Han RQ, Wang PH, Liu AM, Gu X, Zhang XF, Wang XS, Su M, Hu X, Sun Z, Li G, Jin ZY, Jung SY, Mu L, He N, Lu QY, Li L, Zhao JK, Zhang ZF. Raw Garlic Consumption and Risk of Liver Cancer: A Population-Based Case–Control Study in Eastern China. Nutrients. 2019 Aug 31;11(9):2038. http://doi.org/10.3390/nu11092038. PMID: 31480423; PMCID: PMC6769938.

[14] Ngo SN, Williams DB, Cobiac L, Head RJ. Does garlic reduce risk of colorectal cancer? A systematic review. J Nutr. 2007 Oct;137(10):2264–9. http://doi.org/10.1093/jn/137.10.2264. PMID: 17885009.

Yet, clinical trials on human cancer patients are far and few between.[15] In turn, this means that the evidence is encouraging but it is not convincing.

Plausibility	👍
Effectiveness	👎
Safety	👍
Cost	👍
Risk/benefit balance	👎

Glucosamine

Glucosamine is currently one of the most popular of all dietary supplements. It is marketed mostly as a treatment for arthritis, and there is some evidence that it is moderately helpful for this indication. In addition, evidence had been accumulating to suggest that glucosamine might have other positive health effects as well. Several recent epidemiological investigations indicated that glucosamine use might play a role in prevention of cancer.[16 17]

The most recent of these analyses evaluated the associations of regular glucosamine use with all-cause and cause-specific mortality in a large prospective cohort.[18] This population-based prospective cohort study included 495,077 women and men. Participants were recruited from 2006 to 2010 and were followed until 2018. At baseline, 19% of the participants reported regular use of glucosamine supplements. During a median follow-up of 9 years, 19,882 deaths were recorded, including

- 3802 from CVD,

[15] Zhou X, Qian H, Zhang D, Zeng L. Garlic intake and the risk of colorectal cancer: A meta-analysis. *Medicine (Baltimore)*. 2020;99(1):e18575. http://doi.org/10.1097/MD.0000000000018575.

[16] Kantor ED, Lampe JW, Peters U, Shen DD, Vaughan TL, White E. Use of glucosamine and chondroitin supplements and risk of colorectal cancer. *Cancer Causes Control*. 2013;24(6):1137–1146. http://doi.org/10.1007/s10552-013-0192-2.

[17] Ibáñez-Sanz G, Díez-Villanueva A, Vilorio-Marqués L, et al. Possible role of chondroitin sulphate and glucosamine for primary prevention of colorectal cancer. Results from the MCC-Spain study. *Sci Rep*. 2018;8(1):2040. Published 2018 Feb 1. http://doi.org/10.1038/s41598-018-20349-6.

[18] Li ZH, Gao X, Chung VC, et al. Associations of regular glucosamine use with all-cause and cause-specific mortality: a large prospective cohort study. *Ann Rheum Dis*. 2020;79(6):829–836. http://doi.org/10.1136/annrheumdis-2020-217176.

- 8090 from cancer,
- 3380 from respiratory diseases,
- 1061 from digestive diseases.

In multivariable adjusted analyses, the hazard ratios associated with glucosamine use were

- 0.85 (95% CI 0.82 to 0.89) for all-cause mortality,
- 0.82 (95% CI 0.74 to 0.90) for CVD mortality,
- 0.94 (95% CI 0.88 to 0.99) for cancer mortality,
- 0.73 (95% CI 0.66 to 0.81) for respiratory mortality,
- 0.74 (95% CI 0.62 to 0.90) for digestive mortality.

The authors concluded that *regular glucosamine supplementation was associated with lower mortality due to all causes, cancer, CVD, respiratory and digestive diseases.*

It is well documented that glucosamine has powerful anti-inflammatory effects. Therefore it is conceivable that such anti-inflammatory mechanisms are the cause for the observed outcomes. However, at present, the evidence is based mostly on observational data which can be suggestive but not conclusive.

Plausibility	👍
Effectiveness	🤏
Safety	👍
Cost	👍
Risk/benefit balance	🤏

Green Tea

Green tea (*Camellia sinensis*) is the tea made from unfermented tea leaves. It is rich in epigallocatechin gallate (EGCG), also known as epigallocatechin-3-gallate which, in test tubes, inhibits cancer cell proliferation by inducing apoptosis and cell cycle arrest. In addition, EGCG might inhibit tumour cell metastasis and angiogenesis.[19] However, it is worth noting that daily ingestion of more than 800 mg of EGCG has been associated with liver damage.[20]

A Cochrane review of green tea as a preventative of cancer we included in total 142 completed studies (11 experimental and 131 nonexperimental) and two ongoing studies. The authors concluded that the *findings from experimental and nonexperimental epidemiological studies yielded inconsistent results, thus providing limited evidence for the beneficial effect of green tea consumption on the overall risk of cancer or on specific cancer sites. Some evidence of a beneficial effect of green tea at some cancer sites emerged from the RCTs and from case–control studies, but their methodological limitations, such as the low number and size of the studies, and the inconsistencies with the results of cohort studies, limit the interpretability of the RR estimates. The studies also indicated the occurrence of several side effects associated with high intakes of green tea. In addition, the majority of included studies were carried out in Asian populations characterised by a high intake of green tea, thus limiting the generalisability of the findings to other populations. Well conducted and adequately powered RCTs would be needed to draw conclusions on the possible beneficial effects of green tea consumption on cancer risk.*[21] The evidence that green tea consumption is effective as a means of cancer prevention is thus encouraging but not convincing.

Plausibility	👍
Effectiveness	👎
Safety	👎
Cost	👍
Risk/benefit balance	👎

[19] Aggarwal V, Tuli HS, Tania M, Srivastava S, Ritzer EE, Pandey A, Aggarwal D, Barwal TS, Jain A, Kaur G, Sak K, Varol M, Bishayee A. Molecular mechanisms of action of epigallocatechin gallate in cancer: Recent trends and advancement. Semin Cancer Biol. 2020 May 24:S1044-579X(20)30107-3. http://doi.org/10.1016/j.semcancer.2020.05.011. Epub ahead of print. PMID: 32461153.

[20] Dekant W, Fujii K, Shibata E, Morita O, Shimotoyodome A. Safety assessment of green tea based beverages and dried green tea extracts as nutritional supplements. Toxicol Lett. 2017 Aug 5;277:104–108. http://doi.org/10.1016/j.toxlet.2017.06.008. Epub 2017 Jun 24. PMID: 28655517.

[21] Filippini T, Malavolti M, Borrelli F, et al. Green tea (Camellia sinensis) for the prevention of cancer. *Cochrane Database Syst Rev.* 2020;3(3):CD005004. Published 2020 Mar 2. http://doi.org/10.1002/14651858.CD005004.pub3.

Lycopene

Lycopene is the bright red carotenoid found in tomatoes and other red fruits and vegetables, such as red carrots, watermelons, grapefruits, and papayas. It is commonly found in dishes prepared from tomatoes. When it was discovered that lycopene might generate positive health effects, numerous lycopene-containing supplements came on the market.

A systematic review of epidemiological studies concluded that *higher dietary and circulating lycopene concentrations are inversely associated with prostate cancer risk. This was accompanied by dose–response relationships for dietary and circulating lycopene. However, lycopene was not associated with a reduced risk of advanced prostate cancer.*[22] While these data seem encouraging, the evidence from clinical trials is scarce and disappointing.[23]

Plausibility	👍
Effectiveness	🤚
Safety	👍
Cost	👍
Risk/benefit balance	🤚

Phyto-oestrogens

Phyto-oestrogens are non-endocrine, non-steroidal secondary derivatives of plants that have similar actions in the body as oestrogens. The major sources of phyto-oestrogens are soy and soy-based foods, flaxseed (see above), chickpeas, green beans and dairy products. Phyto-oestrogens exert their

[22] Rowles JL 3rd, Ranard KM, Smith JW, An R, Erdman JW Jr. Increased dietary and circulating lycopene are associated with reduced prostate cancer risk: a systematic review and meta-analysis. Prostate Cancer Prostatic Dis. 2017 Dec;20(4):361–377. http://doi.org/10.1038/pcan.2017.25. Epub 2017 Apr 25. PMID: 28440323.

[23] Posadzki P, Lee MS, Onakpoya I, Lee HW, Ko BS, Ernst E. Dietary supplements and prostate cancer: a systematic review of double-blind, placebo-controlled randomised clinical trials. Maturitas. 2013 Jun;75(2):125–30. http://doi.org/10.1016/j.maturitas.2013.03.006. Epub 2013 Apr 6. PMID: 23567264.

effects mainly by binding to the body's oestrogen receptors. They are absorbed in the gut and are said to have a wide range of effects on human health.

Phyto-oestrogens might play an inhibitory role during the initial phases of cancer development. Experimental and physiologic studies have provided some evidence of an inverse association between breast cancer risk and phytoestrogen intake.[24] However, research in humans has been limited to epidemiologic studies and is therefore far from conclusive.

Plausibility	👍
Effectiveness	👎
Safety	👍
Cost	👍
Risk/benefit balance	👎

Probiotics

Probiotics consist of microorganisms claimed to convey health benefits by improving or restoring the gut flora (Sect. 3.4). Changes in the gut microenvironment, such as undesirable changes in the microbiota composition, provide a fertile environment for intestinal inflammation and cancer development. The administration of certain probiotics is said to partly reverse this situation.

Probiotics might influence the development of gastrointestinal cancers by enhancing the immune barrier, regulating the intestinal immune state, inhibiting pathogenic enzyme activity, regulating cancer cell proliferation and apoptosis, regulating redox homeostasis, and reprograming intestinal microbial composition.[25]

A review of the clinical data stated that *the results of many clinical studies indicate the effectiveness of probiotics in preventing, treating and reducing the*

---

[24] Mishra SI, Dickerson V, Najm W. Phytoestrogens and breast cancer prevention: what is the evidence? *Am J Obstet Gynecol*. 2003;188(5 Suppl):S66–S70. http://doi.org/10.1067/mob.2003.405.

[25] Ding S, Hu C, Fang J, Liu G. The Protective Role of Probiotics against Colorectal Cancer. Oxid Med Cell Longev. 2020 Dec 9;2020:8884583. http://doi.org/10.1155/2020/8884583. PMID: 33488940; PMCID: PMC7803265.

progression of several types of cancer including colorectal, liver, breast, bladder, colon, and cervical in cancer patients.[26]

Another review concluded that *studies have provided a theoretical foundation for the roles of probiotics in CRC prevention and treatment, but their mechanisms of action remain to be investigated, and further clinical trials are warranted for the application of probiotics in the target population* (see Footnote 25). Yet another review found that *the alterations of gut microbiota may be used as potential therapeutic approaches to prevent or treat colorectal cancer (CRC). Probiotics such as Lactobacillus and Bifidobacterium inhibit the growth of CRC through inhibiting inflammation and angiogenesis and enhancing the function of the intestinal barrier through the secretion of short-chain fatty acids (SCFAs). Crosstalk between lifestyle, host genetics, and gut microbiota is well documented in the prevention and treatment of CRC.*

Essentially, this indicates that probiotics have considerable potential in the prevention of gastrointestinal and other cancers.

Plausibility	👍
Effectiveness	👍
Safety	👍
Cost	👍
Risk/benefit balance	👍

Selenium

Selenium (Se) is a trace element found in the earth's crust, water and food. It is used industrially, for instance, for making glass and pigments. Selenium is also required for optimal human health; small amounts of selenium are essential for certain biological functions in humans, while higher concentrations are toxic.

Several observational studies reported that people with high levels of selenium in their diet or in their body tissues had lower risk of cancer, and some laboratory studies suggested that selenium inhibits the growth of cancer cells.

[26] Śliżewska K, Markowiak-Kopeć P, Śliżewska W. The Role of Probiotics in Cancer Prevention. Cancers (Basel). 2020 Dec 23;13(1):20. http://doi.org/10.3390/cancers13010020. PMID: 33374549; PMCID: PMC7793079.

In the case–control studies, it was noted that selenium levels in human tissues are negatively correlated with the risk of breast cancer.[27] It was suggested that selenium has anti-cancer properties via acting as an antioxidant.[28]

A 2018 Cochrane review included 83 studies. Its findings showed no beneficial effect of selenium supplements in reducing cancer risk. Some RCTs even reported a higher incidence of high-grade prostate cancer in participants with selenium supplementation. The authors concluded that *overall, there is no evidence to suggest that increasing selenium intake through diet or supplementation prevents cancer in humans.*[29] Thus selenium is not a promising option for cancer prevention.

Plausibility	
Effectiveness	
Safety	
Cost	
Risk/benefit balance	

Various Other Dietary Supplements

A systematic review of the evidence for the use of multivitamins or single nutrients and functionally related nutrient pairs for the primary prevention of cancer generated disappointing findings. The authors included 103 articles representing 26 unique studies.

- Two trials suggested a protective effect of multivitamin supplements against cancer, but only in men.

[27] Zhu X, Pan D, Wang N, Wang S, Sun G. Relationship Between Selenium in Human Tissues and Breast Cancer: a Meta-analysis Based on Case–Control Studies. Biol Trace Elem Res. 2021 Jan 8. http://doi.org/10.1007/s12011-021-02574-9. Epub ahead of print. PMID: 33420696.

[28] Stolwijk JM, Garje R, Sieren JC, Buettner GR, Zakharia Y. Understanding the Redox Biology of Selenium in the Search of Targeted Cancer Therapies. Antioxidants (Basel). 2020 May 13;9(5):420. http://doi.org/10.3390/antiox9050420. PMID: 32414091; PMCID: PMC7278812.

[29] Vinceti M, Filippini T, Del Giovane C, Dennert G, Zwahlen M, Brinkman M, Zeegers MP, Horneber M, D'Amico R, Crespi CM. Selenium for preventing cancer. Cochrane Database Syst Rev. 2018 Jan 29;1(1):CD005195. http://doi.org/10.1002/14651858.CD005195.pub4. PMID: 29376219; PMCID: PMC6491296.

- Beta-carotene showed a negative effect on lung cancer incidence and mortality among individuals at high risk for lung cancer at baseline.
- Vitamin E supplementation yielded mixed results and had no overall effect on cancer or all-cause mortality.
- The few studies addressing folic acid and vitamin A showed no effect on cancer and mortality.
- Vitamin D and/or calcium supplementation also showed no overall effect on cancer and mortality.

The authors' conclusions are less than encouraging: *there is a limited number of trials examining the effects of dietary supplements on … cancer; the majority showed no effect in healthy populations.*[30]

Vegetarian Diet

Vegetarianism is the abstention of meat consumption. It can be adopted for a range of reasons, for instance, ethics, environmental, religion or health. Its strictest form is veganism which rejects all animal products. Vegans can be at risk of vitamin B12 hypovitaminosis and might need supplements.

Many SCAM-proponents assume that a plant-based diet reduces the risk of cancer. However, this assumption is not supported by sound evidence. A systematic review included 26 articles, which were classified into studies on plant-based dietary patterns (PBDPs) and cancer outcomes at pre-diagnosis: vegan/vegetarian diet ($N = 5$), pro-vegetarian diet ($N = 2$), Mediterranean diet ($N = 13$), and studies considering the same at post-diagnosis ($N = 6$). The few studies available on the vegetarian diet failed to support its effectiveness as an effective measure to prevent cancer. The authors concluded that *whether plant-based diets before or after a cancer diagnosis prevent negative cancer-related outcomes needs to be researched further, in order to define dietary guidelines for cancer survivors.*[31]

---

[30] Fortmann SP, Burda BU, Senger CA, Lin JS, Beil TL, O'Connor E, Whitlock EP. Vitamin, Mineral, and Multivitamin Supplements for the Primary Prevention of Cardiovascular Disease and Cancer: A Systematic Evidence Review for the U.S. Preventive Services Task Force [Internet]. Rockville (MD): Agency for Healthcare Research and Quality (US); 2013 Nov. Report No.: 14-05199-EF-1. PMID: 24308073.

[31] Molina-Montes E, Salamanca-Fernández E, Garcia-Villanova B, Sánchez MJ. The Impact of Plant-Based Dietary Patterns on Cancer-Related Outcomes: A Rapid Review and Meta-Analysis. *Nutrients.* 2020;12(7):2010. Published 2020 Jul 6. http://doi.org/10.3390/nu12072010.

Plausibility	👍
Effectiveness	👍
Safety	👍
Cost	👍
Risk/benefit balance	👍

Vitamin C

Vitamin C or ascorbic acid is found in fruit and vegetables and many other foods. People who are healthy and consume a normal diet usually get enough vitamin C and thus need no supplements. Severe vitamin C deficiency is the cause of scurvy and can be cured with vitamin C. Contrary to common belief, vitamin C supplementation is not useful for the prevention of any other condition.

A 2017 systematic review assessed the efficacy of all types of dietary supplements in the primary prevention of cause-specific death, including cancer. Its authors found no important effect of vitamin C on cancer prevention. They concluded that there is *insufficient evidence to support the use of dietary supplements in the primary prevention of … cancer.*[32]

Plausibility	👍
Effectiveness	👎
Safety	👍
Cost	👍
Risk/benefit balance	👎

[32] Schwingshackl L, Boeing H, Stelmach-Mardas M, Gottschald M, Dietrich S, Hoffmann G, Chaimani A. Dietary Supplements and Risk of Cause-Specific Death, Cardiovascular Disease, and Cancer: A Systematic Review and Meta-Analysis of Primary Prevention Trials. Adv Nutr. 2017 Jan 17;8(1):27–39. http://doi.org/10.3945/an.116.013516. PMID: 28096125; PMCID: PMC5227980.

Conclusion

Overall, the belief that SCAM plays a major role in the prevention of cancer is built more on wishful thinking than on strong evidence. The available evidence rests mostly on observational studies which cannot establish cause and effect (Sect. 1.7). Data from clinical trials are scarce and therefore unconvincing. Finally, some of the evidence suggests that some dietary supplements could even have a negative influence.

The best advice for consumers who want to minimise their cancer risk is to eat a balanced diet, to not smoke, to avoid excesses of any kind and to observe the other lifestyle behaviours mentioned above. Should one day any type of SCAM be proven to prevent cancer, it will automatically become a conventional approach. An alternative cancer preventative is, therefore, a contradiction in terms.

3

Alternative Cancer Cures

This chapter is dedicated to those forms of SCAM that are regularly being promoted as alternative cancer cures or treatments that prolong the life of cancer patients, i.e. SCAMs which are claimed to change the natural history of cancer. Changing the natural history means improving the prognosis either by eliminating the cancer completely or by slowing (or accelerating) cancer growth and thus prolonging (or shortening) the life of a cancer patient beyond the statistical average.

There are hundreds, if not thousands of SCAMs that are promoted in this way. It is therefore not possible to deal with all of them here. Instead, I will focus on those SCAMs that are most popular - usually because they are aggressively marketed.

3.1 Plant-Derived 'Natural' Remedies

Herbal medicines are based on extracts of plants or parts of plants (Fig. 3.1). They always contain more than one ingredient. Several such plant-derived ingredients have in the past provided the basis for the development of conventional cancer drugs; examples are Taxol (derived from the yew tree) or Vincristine (derived from the periwinkle). Further plant-derived cancer drugs will unquestionably emerge in the near future. However, like Taxol or Vincristine, they will not belong to the realm of herbal medicine which is defined as the treatment with remedies from whole plants with all its multiple constituents.

© The Author(s), under exclusive license to Springer Nature
Switzerland AG 2021
E. Ernst, *So-Called Alternative Medicine (SCAM) for Cancer*,
https://doi.org/10.1007/978-3-030-74158-7_3

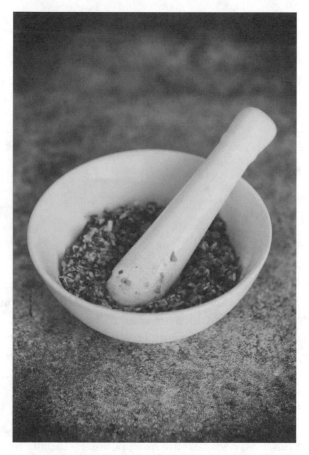

Fig. 3.1 There are thousands of plants traditionally used as medicines; only relatively few have been well researched, and even fewer have been shown to be effective

In this chapter, I will discuss SCAMs that are plant-derived and thus usually considered to be 'natural' herbal remedies, even if this is not always true.

Black Salve

Black salve is a paste for external use made from variable mixtures of herbal and non-herbal ingredients. They usually contain bloodroot and/or chaparral and/or zinc chloride all of which render the products corrosive. This means black salve destroys living cells, and the assumption is that, by applying it to skin cancer, black salve would destroy the tumour and cure the cancer.

Black salve is said to originate from Native American tribes who used the paste as a treatment for a range of conditions. It was adopted by conventional medicine about a century ago as a treatment for several skin problems. When effective treatments became available, black salve became obsolete. More recently, however, it has been re-discovered by SCAM-practitioners who recommend it as a natural treatment for various skin conditions, including cancer.

The available evidence fails to support the assumption that black salve is a cancer cure. No compelling data exist to show that it is efficacious for any condition, especially not for skin cancer, the indication for which it is often promoted. Rigorous clinical trials testing its efficacy are not available. A recent review of the evidence concluded that *black salve is not a natural therapy. It contains significant concentrations of synthetic chemicals. Black salve does not appear to possess tumour specificity with in vitro and in vivo evidence indicating normal cell toxicity. Black salve does appear to cure some skin cancers, although the cure rate for this therapy is currently unknown. The use of black salve should be restricted to clinical research in low-risk malignancies located at low-risk sites until a better understanding of its efficacy and toxicity is developed. Where a therapy capable of harm is already being used by patients, it is ethically irresponsible not to study and analyse its effects. Although cautionary tales are valuable, black salve research needs to move beyond the case study and into the carefully designed clinical trial arena. Only then can patients be properly informed of its true benefits and hazards.*[1]

Due to its erosive nature, black salve burns away the tissue with which it comes into contact. Numerous case reports of the resulting deformations have been published.[2] [3] Many horrendous pictures of patients maimed by their use of black salve can be seen on the Internet and give a dramatic impression of the harm caused. Black salve should be regarded as unsafe.[4]

Plausibility	👎
Effectiveness	👎
Safety	👎

(continued)

[1] Croaker A, King GJ, Pyne JH, Anoopkumar-Dukie S, Liu L. A Review of Black Salve: Cancer Specificity, Cure, and Cosmesis. Evid Based Complement Alternat Med. 2017;2017:9184034. http://doi.org/10.1155/2017/9184034.

[2] Ong NC, Sham E, Adams BM. Use of unlicensed black salve for cutaneous malignancy. Med J Aust. 2014;200(6):314. http://doi.org/10.5694/mja14.00041.

[3] Saltzberg F, Barron G, Fenske N. Deforming self-treatment with herbal "black salve". Dermatol Surg. 2009;35(7):1152–1154. http://doi.org/10.1111/j.1524-4725.2009.01206.x.

[4] Lim A. Black salve treatment of skin cancer: a review. J Dermatolog Treat. 2018;29(4):388–392. http://doi.org/10.1080/09546634.2017.1395795.

(continued)

Cost	
Risk/benefit balance	

Cannabis

The genus Cannabis (or marijuana) belongs to the *cannabaceae* family and has been traditionally used as medicinal plant against diseases such as asthma, malaria, treatment of skin diseases, diabetes, and headache. Cannabis has anti-bacterial, anti-fungal, and anti-inflammatory properties. Its modern medicinal indications are mainly pain, epilepsy and cancer.

Different cannabis compounds have different actions; as single compounds, they are not strictly speaking herbal remedies. Delta-9-tetrahydrocannabinol (THC) causes the "high" reported by recreational marijuana users. THC can also help relieve pain and nausea of cancer patients. Cannabidiol (CBD) treats epilepsy and can reduce anxiety or paranoia. CBD oils contain only small amounts of THC. Cancer patients often use CBD for a variety of conditions, particularly pain and nausea, without experiencing the intoxicating adverse effects of marijuana.

Cannabis oil is also being recommended as a cure for various cancers. Cannabinoids have been shown to reduce the size of prostate cancer tumours in animal models.[5] Isolated case reports have yielded encouraging findings also in human cancers, for instance, in acute lymphoblastic leukaemia.[6] However, case reports cannot be considered to be reliable evidence (Sect. 1.7), and there are currently no data from rigorous clinical trials to suggest that cannabis products will alter the natural history of any cancer.[7]

Plausibility	

(continued)

[5] Singh K, Jamshidi N, Zomer R, Piva TJ, Mantri N. Cannabinoids and Prostate Cancer: A Systematic Review of Animal Studies. *Int J Mol Sci*. 2020;21(17):E6265. Published 2020 Aug 29. http://doi.org/10.3390/ijms21176265.

[6] Singh Y, Bali C. Cannabis extract treatment for terminal acute lymphoblastic leukemia with a Philadelphia chromosome mutation. *Case Rep Oncol*. 2013;6(3):585–592. Published 2013 Nov 28. http://doi.org/10.1159/000356446.

[7] Abu-Amna M, Salti T, Khoury M, Cohen I, Bar-Sela G. Medical Cannabis in Oncology: a Valuable Unappreciated Remedy or an Undesirable Risk? Curr Treat Options Oncol. 2021 Jan 13;22(2):16. http://doi.org/10.1007/s11864-020-00811-2. PMID: 33439370.

(continued)

Effectiveness	👎
Safety	👍
Cost	👎
Risk/benefit balance	👎

Carctol

Carctol is a herbal mixture designed by Dr. Nandlal Tiwari, an Ayurvedic practitioner who claims it cures all types of cancer at all stages of the disease, even when conventional treatments have failed. One capsule of Carctol contains Hemidesmus indicus root, Tribulus terrestris seeds, Piper cubeba Linn. Seeds, Ammani vesicatoria plant, Lepidium sativum Linn. Seeds, Blepharis edulis seeds, Smilax china Linn. Roots, Rheumemodi wall roots.[8]

Several promotional websites claim that 30–40% of all patients will respond to Carctol therapy. As Carctol is said to act slowly, cancer patients are instructed to take it for several months. The total costs for this treatment are therefore considerable. Tiwari claims that Carctol depletes the body of acidity creating an alkaline environment which, in turn, kills cancer cells. There is, however, no evidence that this is true. In fact, no good evidence exists to show that Carctol helps cancer patients in any way.[9]

Plausibility	👎
Effectiveness	👎
Safety	👎
Cost	👎
Risk/benefit balance	👎

[8] https://www.carctol.in/about.html.
[9] Ernst E. Carctol: Profit before Patients?. *Breast Care (Basel).* 2009;4(1):31–33. http://doi.org/10.1159/000193025.

Chinese Herbal Mixtures

Chinese herbal medicine has a very long tradition which prompts many enthusiasts to assume it has 'stood the test of time'. This assumption is, however, little more than a logical fallacy and, despite a plethora of (mostly seriously flawed) research, both its risks and its benefits remain uncertain. Practitioners of Chinese herbal medicine usually employ mixtures that contain a multitude of different plants. As every single plant already contains numerous ingredients, such mixtures are chaotically complex. The ancient Chinese literature recorded more than 100,000 recipes, some of which also contain non-botanical ingredients, like minerals or animal parts.

Clinical trials of Chinese herbal mixtures are mostly published in Chinese, and there are several reasons for being sceptical about their reliability; fraud seems to be rife,[10] and Chinese researchers publish almost nothing but positive results.[11] Another major problem is the often dismal methodological quality of the primary studies. A systematic review of almost 2385 RCTs of TCM treatments for cancer, for instance, showed that only 394 of them had adequate descriptions on the randomisation method, and only 63 included blinding.[12]

A plethora of reviews of these studies have recently become available also in English. The conclusions are usually encouraging, however, because the primary studies' lack of reliability, caution is advised. Here are the abstracts of just two examples:

This study aimed to compare the efficacy and safety of traditional Chinese medicines (TCMs) combined with paclitaxel-based chemotherapy and paclitaxel-based chemotherapy alone for gastric cancer treatment. Literature searches (up to September 25, 2019) were performed using the Cochrane Library, EMBASE, PubMed, Chinese Science and Technology Journals (CQVIP), Wanfang, and China Academic Journals (CNKI) databases. Data from 14 randomized controlled trials (RCTs), with 1109 participants, were included. The results indicated that, compared with paclitaxel-based chemotherapy alone, the combination of TCMs and paclitaxel-based chemotherapy significantly improved the tumour response rate (TRR; RR: 1.39; 95% CI: 1.24–1.57; $p < 0.001$, I2 $=$ 12%), increased the quality of life

---

[10] https://www.rfa.org/english/news/china/clinical-fakes-09272016141438.html.

[11] Tang JL, Zhan SY, Ernst E. Review of randomised controlled trials of traditional Chinese medicine. *BMJ*. 1999;319(7203):160–161. http://doi.org/10.1136/bmj.319.7203.160.

[12] Li X, Yang G, Li X, et al. Traditional Chinese medicine in cancer care: a review of controlled clinical studies published in chinese, published correction appears in PLoS One. 2013;8(6). http://doi.org/10.1371/annotation/b53a0b8b-3eb6-44a2-9c37-bc9bb66bfe7e. *PLoS One*. 2013;8(4):e60338. http://doi.org/10.1371/journal.pone.0060338.

based on the Karnofsky Performance Scale score (RR: 1.53; 95% CI: 1.19–1.96; $p < 0.001$, I2 = 0%), and reduced the side effects, such as neutropenia (RR: 0.68; 95% CI: 0.55–0.84; $p < 0.001$, I2 = 44%), leukopenia (RR: 0.69; 95% CI: 0.54–0.90; $p < 0.01$, I2 = 40%), thrombocytopenia (RR: 0.66; 95% CI: 0.46–0.96; $p < 0.05$, I2 = 32%), and nausea and vomiting (RR: 0.50; 95% CI: 0.32–0.80; $p < 0.01$, I2 = 85%). Hepatic dysfunction (RR: 0.63; 95% CI: 0.33–1.20; $p = 0.16$, I2 = 0%), neurotoxicity (RR: 0.64; 95% CI: 0.26–1.55; $p = 0.32$, I2 = 0%), and anemia (RR: 0.65; 95% CI: 0.40–1.04; $p = 0.07$, I2 = 0%) were similar between the two groups. Evidence from the meta-analysis suggested that compared with paclitaxel-based chemotherapy alone, the combination of TCMs and paclitaxel-based chemotherapy may increase the TRR, improve quality of life, and reduce multiple chemotherapy-related side effects in gastric cancer patients. Additional rigorously designed large RCTs are required to confirm the efficacy and safety of this treatment.[13]

This meta analysis evaluated the comparative safety and efficacy for the addition of Astragalus-based Chinese medicines combined with chemotherapy and chemotherapy alone for colorectal cancer (CRC) treatment. Systematic literature search was performed by PubMed, EMBSAE, Ovid, Web of Science, Cochrane Library, Chinese Science and Technology Journals (CQVIP), China Academic Journals (CNKI), and Chinese Biomedical Literature database. A total of 22 studies which reported on 1,409 subjects were identified. This meta-analysis indicated that the combination of Astragalus-based Chinese medicines and chemotherapy may increase the efficiency of tumour response rate (TRR) for the treatment of CRC patients (RR: 1.52; 95% CI: 1.24–1.87; $p < 0.0001$), improve their life quality based on KPS (RR: 2.51; 95% CI: 1.85–3.42; $p < 0.00001$ and WMD: 10.96; 95% CI: 9.45–12.47; $p < 0.00001$), and reduce the adverse reactions, including neutropenia (RR: 0.52; 95% CI: 0.44–0.62; $p < 0.00001$), anemia (RR: 0.49; 95% CI: 0.34–0.70; $p < 0.0001$), thrombocytopenia (RR: 0.59; 95% CI: 0.46–0.77; $p = 0.0001$), nausea and vomiting (RR: 0.56; 95% CI: 0.46–0.68; $p < 0.00001$), diarrhea (RR: 0.55; 95% CI: 0.40–0.75; $p = 0.0001$), and neurotoxicity (RR: 0.56; 95% CI: 0.49–0.65; $p < 0.00001$). Hepatic dysfunction (RR: 0.76; 95% CI: 0.53–1.09; $p = 0.13$) and renal dysfunction (RR: 0.95; 95% CI: 0.51–1.76; $p = 0.87$) were similar between two groups. The results showed that Astragalus-based Chinese medicines combined with chemotherapy in the treatment of CRC may increase

---

[13] Li Y, Sui X, Su Z, et al. Meta-Analysis of Paclitaxel-Based Chemotherapy Combined With Traditional Chinese Medicines for Gastric Cancer Treatment. *Front Pharmacol*. 2020;11:132. Published 2020 Feb 27. http://doi.org/10.3389/fphar.2020.00132.

the efficiency of TRR, reduce chemotherapeutic agents-associated adverse reactions, and improve their life quality when compared with chemotherapy alone, but further randomized studies are warranted.[14]

Such reviews tell us very little about the true value of Chinese herbal mixtures. They are based on poor-quality studies, lack critical evaluation of the primary data and arrive at over-optimistic conclusions. As such, these reviews can mislead vulnerable cancer patients into making regrettable choices.

It would, of course, not be surprising if researchers one day identified molecules in plants used in Chinese herbal medicine that can be developed into effective cancer treatments. At present, however, there is no convincing evidence that Chinese herbal remedies are effective cancer cures and a plethora of evidence to indicate that they may cause harm.

Plausibility	👍
Effectiveness	👎
Safety	👎
Cost	👎
Risk/benefit balance	👎

Curcumin

Curcumin (turmeric) is the active component in turmeric (*Curcuma longa*). As turmeric is a well known Asian spice that has been used for millennia, it is generally considered to be safe. Several in vitro and in vivo studies have suggested that curcumin has antiproliferative, antiangiogenic, and apoptotic properties. Consequently, curcumin is often recommended as a cancer cure by SCAM practitioners, particularly after the publication of a widely reported paper entitled '*Long-term stabilisation of myeloma with curcumin*'.[15] But a case report does, of course, not constitute convincing evidence (Sect. 1.7); the question is what do the results from robust clinical trials tell us?

---

[14] Lin S, An X, Guo Y, et al. Meta-Analysis of Astragalus-Containing Traditional Chinese Medicine Combined With Chemotherapy for Colorectal Cancer: Efficacy and Safety to Tumor Response. *Front Oncol.* 2019;9:749. Published 2019 Aug 13. http://doi.org/10.3389/fonc.2019.00749.

[15] Zaidi A, Lai M, Cavenagh J. Long-term stabilisation of myeloma with curcumin. *BMJ Case Rep.* 2017;2017:bcr2016218148. Published 2017 Apr 16. http://doi.org/10.1136/bcr-2016-218148.

- One placebo-controlled RCT included 97 prostate cancer patients and concluded that *six months' intake of oral curcumin did not significantly affect the overall off-treatment duration of intermittent androgen deprivation. However, PSA elevation was suppressed with curcumin intake during the curcumin administration period. Curcumin at this dose was well-tolerated and safe.*[16]
- In another study, 150 women with advanced and metastatic breast cancer were randomly assigned to receive either the conventional drug paclitaxel plus placebo or paclitaxel plus curcumin intravenously for 12 weeks with 3 months of follow-up. The results showed that *curcumin in combination with paclitaxel was superior to the paclitaxel-placebo combination with respect to objective response rate and physical performance after 12 weeks of treatment.*[17]
- In a trial of 44 patients with familial adenomatous polyposis, no difference was found in the mean number or size of lower intestinal tract adenomas (considered to be pre-cancerous lesions) between patients given curcumin 3000 mg/day and those given placebo for 12 weeks.[18]

Curcumin does undoubtedly have promising pharmacological activities and has thus become widely used.[19] Research into curcumin is highly active to solve the existing problems such as curcumin's low bioavailability after oral administration. Consequently, preparations of curcumin might one day become useful cancer drugs. As such they would, however, be conventional medicines and could no longer be considered a SCAM (see above). For the time being, curcumin cannot be considered to be a demonstrably effective cure for any cancer.

Plausibility	👍
Effectiveness	👎

(continued)

[16] Choi YH, Han DH, Kim SW, et al. A randomized, double-blind, placebo-controlled trial to evaluate the role of curcumin in prostate cancer patients with intermittent androgen deprivation. *Prostate.* 2019;79(6):614–621. http://doi.org/10.1002/pros.23766.

[17] Saghatelyan T, Tananyan A, Janoyan N, et al. Efficacy and safety of curcumin in combination with paclitaxel in patients with advanced, metastatic breast cancer: A comparative, randomized, double-blind, placebo-controlled clinical trial [published online ahead of print, 2020 Apr 18]. *Phytomedicine.* 2020;70:153218. http://doi.org/10.1016/j.phymed.2020.153218.

[18] Cruz-Correa M, Hylind LM, Marrero JH, et al. Efficacy and Safety of Curcumin in Treatment of Intestinal Adenomas in Patients With Familial Adenomatous Polyposis. *Gastroenterology.* 2018;155(3):668–673. http://doi.org/10.1053/j.gastro.2018.05.031.

[19] Tas F, Cinar E, Erturk K. Complementary and alternative medicine (CAM) in Turkish cutaneous melanoma patients: A prospective study from tertiary cancer center. J Oncol Pharm Pract. 2021 Jan 12:1078155220987637. http://doi.org/10.1177/1078155220987637. Epub ahead of print. PMID: 33435821.

(continued)

Safety	👍
Cost	👍
Risk/benefit balance	👎

Danshen

Danshen (*Radix Salviae Miltiorrhizae*) is a herbal remedy that is part of many Chinese herbal mixtures (see above) and has allegedly been used in clinical practice for over 2000 years. It is often recommended as a cancer cure. The active ingredients of Danshen seem to be 15,16-dihydrotanshinone (DHT) which is said to have anti-cancer, cardiovascular, anti-inflammation, anti-Alzheimer and other effects.[20]

A systematic review evaluated the evidence for Danshen as a treatment of cancer. Thirteen RCTs with a total of 1045 participants were included. The studies investigated lung cancer ($n = 5$), leukaemia ($n = 3$), liver cancer ($n = 3$), breast or colon cancer ($n = 1$), and gastric cancer ($n = 1$). The meta-analysis suggested that Danshen formulae had a significant effect on the response rate, 1-year survival, 3-year survival, and 5-year survival. The authors concluded that *the current research results showed that Danshen formulae combined with chemotherapy for cancer treatment was better than conventional drug treatment plan alone.*[21] While these findings seem promising, it is important to stress that this review has several limitations:

- Most of the included studies were of poor quality.
- The trials used 83 different herbal mixtures of variable quality containing Danshen. It is therefore not possible to define precisely which ingredients in the mixtures worked and which did not.
- There is no discussion of the adverse effects and no mention of possible herb-drug interactions.
- The review is wide open to publication bias.

---

[20] Chen X, Yu J, Zhong B, Lu J, Lu JJ, Li S, Lu Y. Pharmacological activities of dihydrotanshinone I, a natural product from Salvia miltiorrhiza Bunge. Pharmacol Res. 2019 July;145:104254. http://doi.org/10.1016/j.phrs.2019.104254. Epub 2019 May 1. PMID: 31054311.

[21] Wang T, Fu X, Wang Z. Danshen Formulae for Cancer: A Systematic Review and Meta-Analysis of High-Quality Randomized Controlled Trials. Evid Based Complement Alternat Med. 2019 Apr 2;2019:2310639. http://doi.org/10.1155/2019/2310639. PMID: 31061667; PMCID: PMC6466905.

- All the primary studies were conducted in China and, as mentioned before, such trials tend to be unreliable.[22]

What follows is simple: it might be that DHT can be developed into a useful drug,[23] however, the notion that Danshen is an effective cancer cure is not supported by sound evidence.

Plausibility	👍
Effectiveness	👎
Safety	👍
Cost	👍
Risk/benefit balance	👎

Essiac

Essiac is a herbal mixture invented by the Canadian nurse Rene Caisse (1888–1978) in the 1920s. The remedy has been promoted as an alternative cancer cure ever since. Caisse stated that she received the formula for Essiac by one of her patients, a claim that has never been independently verified. Essiac is taken as a tea and contains 4 herbal ingredients, but its precise formula is a secret.

There is no good evidence to suggest that Essiac cures any form of cancer. A Canadian study showed no clear evidence of improvement in survival of cancer patients taking Essiac. The Canadian government reviewed the cases of 86 cancer patients who had taken Essiac and reported that it was not clear, if any changes in their conditions had been caused by Essiac.[24] A 2015 review concluded that there is a lack of both safety and efficacy data for Essiac.[25]

---

[22] https://edzardernst.com/2016/10/data-fabrication-in-china-is-an-open-secret/.

[23] Wang X, Yang Y, Liu X, Gao X. Pharmacological properties of tanshinones, the natural products from Salvia miltiorrhiza. Adv Pharmacol. 2020;87:43–70. http://doi.org/10.1016/bs.apha.2019.10.001. Epub 2020 Jan 13. PMID: 32089238.

[24] Essiac/Flor Essence (PDQ®) Patient Version, PDQ Integrative, Alternative, and Complementary Therapies Editorial Board. Published online: December 11, 2015. https://www.ncbi.nlm.nih.gov/books/NBK66020/.

[25] Ulbricht C, Weissner W, Hashmi S, et al. Essiac: systematic review by the natural standard research collaboration. *J Soc Integr Oncol*. 2009;7(2):73–80.

All attempts to get Essiac and related products registered as anti-cancer drugs have failed. Today, Essiac is marketed as a dietary supplement by numerous companies which all produce similar or identical preparations.

Plausibility	👎
Effectiveness	👎
Safety	👎
Cost	👍
Risk/benefit balance	👎

Laetrile

Laetrile is a semisynthetic version of amygdalin which is a compound found in the kernels of apricots and parts of other plants. It is usually administered by mouth as a pill or, less commonly, by injection. Laetrile has been promoted since the 1930s as an alternative cancer cure (Fig. 3.2), but no anti-cancer effects have been shown in clinical trials. The current Cochrane review concluded that *the claims that laetrile or amygdalin have beneficial effects for cancer patients are not currently supported by sound clinical data. There is a considerable risk of serious adverse effects from cyanide poisoning after laetrile or amygdalin, especially after oral ingestion. The risk–benefit balance of laetrile or amygdalin as a treatment for cancer is therefore unambiguously negative.*[26]

Laetrile can cause serious adverse effects. Yet, it has remained popular and even some cancer charities promote it: *Laetrile is a non-toxic extract of apricot kernels. The claimed mechanism of action that is broken down by enzymes found in cancer cells. Hydrogen cyanide, one of the products of this reaction then has a local toxic effect on the cells.*[27] Such misleading promotion of useless and harmful SCAMs is irresponsible and highlights the need for evidence-based information in this area.

[26] Milazzo S, Horneber M. Laetrile treatment for cancer. *Cochrane Database Syst Rev.* 2015;2015(4):CD005476. Published 2015 Apr 28. http://doi.org/10.1002/14651858.CD005476.pub4.

[27] http://yestolife.org.uk/all_therapies.php.

LAETRILE WARNING

Cancer patients and their families are warned that:

LAETRILE IS WORTHLESS

Whether sold as a drug (amygdalin) or as a "vitamin" (B-17), Laetrile is worthless in the prevention, treatment or cure of cancer. The substance has no therapeutic or nutritional value.

LAETRILE IS DANGEROUS

Laetrile can be fatal for cancer patients who delay or give up regular medical treatment and take Laetrile instead.

Laetrile contains cyanide and can cause poisoning and death when taken by mouth. One infant is known dead of cyanide poisoning after swallowing fewer than five Laetrile tablets. At least 16 other deaths have been documented from ingestion of Laetrile ingredients (apricot and similar fruit pits).

Laetrile is especially hazardous if the injection form is taken by mouth. This can cause sudden death.

LAETRILE MAY BE CONTAMINATED

Laetrile is not routinely subject to FDA inspection for quality and purity as are all other drugs.
Analysis has shown some Laetrile to contain toxic contaminants. Ampules of Laetrile for injection have been found with mold and other adulterants which can be dangerous when injected.

Those who persist in the use of Laetrile or its ingredients should:

• Be prepared to deal promptly with acute cyanide poisoning if the oral product is used. Vigorous medical treatment must be started immediately or death can result.

• Watch for early symptoms of chronic cyanide poisoning, including weakness in the arms and legs and disorders of the nervous system.

• Keep the drug out of reach of children.

GET THE FACTS

For full details about the hazards of Laetrile, see your family physician or a cancer specialist, or write the Food and Drug Administration, Laetrile, HFG-20, 5600 Fishers Lane, Rockville, Maryland 20857.

Donald Kennedy
Commissioner of Food and Drugs

Fig. 3.2 FDA warning about Laetrile from 1931. *Source* US National Library of Medicine

Plausibility	
Effectiveness	

(continued)

(continued)

Safety	👎
Cost	👎
Risk/benefit balance	👎

Misteltoe

Mistletoe (*Viscum album*) is a semi-parasitic plant that lives on trees such as oak, elm, pine and apple. Its use as cancer treatment goes back to Rudolf Steiner (1861–1925), the founder of anthroposophical medicine. Steiner considered that mistletoe lives off its host tree much like a cancer lives from a patient's body; in both cases, the eventual outcome is often the death of the host. Following the 'like cures like' assumption of homeopathy, Steiner assumed that mistletoe might be an effective cancer cure and developed his mistletoe preparation, 'Iscador', marketed by Weleda, a firm founded by a collaborator of Steiner.

Iscador is a fermented mistletoe extract and still the most widely used mistletoe product. Some test-tube experiments suggest that ingredients of mistletoe might indeed have anti-cancer activities.[28] The two main therapeutic claims for mistletoe remedies are that:

- they can cure cancer,
- they improve the quality of life of cancer patients.

These claims have been tested in numerous clinical trials most of which are of poor quality.

- A systematic review concluded *that none of the methodologically stronger trials exhibited efficacy in terms of quality of life, survival or other outcome measures. Rigorous trials of mistletoe extracts fail to demonstrate efficacy of this therapy.*[29]

---

[28] Yau T, Dan X, Ng CC, Ng TB. Lectins with potential for anti-cancer therapy. Molecules. 2015 Feb 26;20(3):3791–810. http://doi.org/10.3390/molecules20033791. PMID: 25730388; PMCID: PMC6272365.

[29] Ernst E, Schmidt K, Steuer-Vogt MK. Mistletoe for cancer? A systematic review of randomised clinical trials. Int J Cancer. 2003 Nov 1;107(2):262–7. http://doi.org/10.1002/ijc.11386. PMID: 12949804.

- Another review found that *there was no difference in survival or quality of life measures in patients who received mistletoe compared to those who did not.*[30]
- And a Cochrane review concluded that *the evidence from RCTs to support the view that the application of mistletoe extracts has impact on survival or leads to an improved ability to fight cancer or to withstand anticancer treatments is weak. Nevertheless, there is some evidence that mistletoe extracts may offer benefits on measures of QOL during chemotherapy for breast cancer, but these results need replication. Overall, more high quality, independent clinical research is needed to truly assess the safety and effectiveness of mistletoe extracts. Patients receiving mistletoe therapy should be encouraged to take part in future trails.*[31]

Mistletoe injections are not free of side effects, and have been associated with soreness, inflammation at the injection site, headache, fever, and chills. Contrary to many claims to the opposite, there is no good evidence to suggest that mistletoe is an effective cancer therapy.

Plausibility	👎
Effectiveness	👎
Safety	👎
Cost	👎
Risk/benefit balance	👎

Reishi

Reishi (*Ganoderma lucidum*) is a mushroom that grows in Asia and has been used in Traditional Chinese Medicine for thousands of years. It contains polysaccharides, triterpeniods, proteins and amino acids which are claimed to be responsible for its alleged anti-cancer and immunostimulatory effects.

[30] Mistletoe Extracts (PDQ®), Patient Version, PDQ Integrative, Alternative, and Complementary Therapies Editorial Board. Published online: August 18, 2020.

[31] Horneber MA, Bueschel G, Huber R, Linde K, Rostock M. Mistletoe therapy in oncology. Cochrane Database Syst Rev. 2008 Apr 16;2008(2):CD003297. http://doi.org/10.1002/14651858.CD003297.pub2. PMID: 18425885; PMCID: PMC7144832.

Since several laboratory studies have suggested anti-cancer and other effects, its popularity as an alternative cancer cure has been increasing.

Yet, a Cochrane review *did not find sufficient evidence to justify the use of G. lucidum as a first-line treatment for cancer. It remains uncertain whether G. lucidum helps prolong long-term cancer survival.*[32] Reishi is generally well tolerated and has been associated with only minor adverse events. As it interacts with several conventional drugs, caution is nevertheless advised.

Plausibility	👍
Effectiveness	👎
Safety	👍
Cost	👍
Risk/benefit balance	👎

Ukrain

Ukrain is a semi-synthetic medicine derived from greater celandine (*Chelidonium majus*) and marketed by Vasyl Novytskyi. It contains alkaloids and thiophosphoric acid. The UK charity 'Yes to Life' advertises Ukrain stating that it is *a type of low toxicity chemotherapy derived from a combination of two known cytotoxic drugs that are of little use individually, as the doses required for effective anticancer action are too high to be tolerated. However, the combination is effective at far lower doses, with few side effects.*[33]

Such claims are, however, highly misleading. A systematic review of the clinical trials of Ukrain concluded that *the data from randomised clinical trials suggest Ukrain to have potential as an anticancer drug. However, numerous caveats prevent a positive conclusion, and independent rigorous studies are urgently needed.*[34] Since then, no further convincing evidence has emerged.

---

[32] Jin X, Ruiz Beguerie J, Sze DM, Chan GC. Ganoderma lucidum (Reishi mushroom) for cancer treatment. Cochrane Database Syst Rev. 2016 Apr 5;4(4):CD007731. http://doi.org/10.1002/146 51858.CD007731.pub3. PMID: 27045603; PMCID: PMC6353236.

[33] http://yestolife.org.uk/all_therapies.php.

[34] Ernst E, Schmidt K. Ukrain. A new cancer cure? A systematic review of randomised clinical trials. BMC Cancer. 2005 July 1;5:69. http://doi.org/10.1186/1471-2407-5-69. PMID: 15992405; PMCID: PMC1180428.

Adverse effects include injection site reactions, slight fever, fatigue, dizziness, nausea, and possibly tumour bleeding. Based on the best evidence available to date, Ukrain cannot be categorised as an effective cancer cure.

Plausibility	👎
Effectiveness	👎
Safety	👎
Cost	👎
Risk/benefit balance	👎

Other Alternative Cancer Cures

As already mentioned, there are many SCAMs promoted as alternative cancer cures based on plants. The following list is therefore far from complete, but merely provides a flavour of the range and confusion that cancer patients are exposed to

- Cats claw (*Uncaria tomentosa*) allegedly stimulates the immune system and thus inhibits tumour growth. There is no good evidence that it cures cancer.
- Chaparral (*Larrea tridentata*) originates from American Indians. It is consumed as tea and claimed to suppress cancer cell proliferation. There is no good evidence that it cures cancer.
- Esberitox is a German remedy composed of several herbs, Vitamin C and other ingredients. It allegedly prevents leukopenia during cancer treatment. There is no good evidence that it cures cancer.
- Ginseng is supposed to stimulate the immune system and inhibit cancer progression. There is no good evidence that it cures cancer.
- Haelan 951 is a drink made of fermented soy proteins. It is claimed to stimulate the immune system and slow tumour growth. There is no good evidence that it cures cancer.
- Indol-3-carbinol is a chemical from broccoli supposed to treat hormone-dependent cancers. There is no good evidence that it cures cancer.
- Maitake is a mushroom frequently used in TCM and supposed to stimulate immune defence. There is no good evidence that it cures cancer.

- Noni (*Morinda citrifolia*) originates from Polynesian medicine and is alleged to inhibit tumour growth. There is no good evidence that it cures cancer.
- PC-Spes is a herbal mixture specifically promoted as a cure for prostate cancer. There is no good evidence that it cures cancer.
- Shitake is a mushroom frequently used in TCM and supposed to stimulate immune defence. There is no good evidence that it cures cancer.

None of the remedies on the list have been shown to be effective cancer cures.

Plausibility	👎
Effectiveness	👎
Safety	👎
Cost	👎
Risk/benefit balance	👎

Comment

These examples of commonly used plant-derived cancer cures reveal several common and concerning features. Despite the fact that they are not supported by robust evidence of effectiveness, they remain popular, in some cases even for decades. This is due mainly to intensive and clever marketing and promotion, further aided by the conspiracy theory that 'the establishment' is trying to suppress SCAM (Chap. 6). As mentioned above, even some cancer charities are involved in misleading cancer patients into believing that these 'natural cures' are worth trying.

Often the only evidence for plant-derived cancer cures stems from test tube experiments. To a lay person, it may well sound impressive that a plant extract kills cancer cells in vitro. However, it is neither unusual nor necessarily meaningful. Many plants have such 'anti-cancer' activity but turn out to be far too toxic, too weak, too poorly absorbed, etc. to be of any clinical use.

As research into this area continues, some ingredients of plants might well turn out to become effective cancer treatments. This has happened before, for instance with Taxol, and it will happen again. It is important to note that, when it does, the result will be a conventional cancer drug and not a

SCAM. Single-molecule medicines are not herbal remedies, even if they were originally derived from a plant.

Plant-based alternative cancer cures often command a high retail price, and the profit margins for the entrepreneurs who market them are attractive. Cancer patients are frequently desperate and easy prey for those who sell false hope at exorbitant prices. Personally, I can imagine only few things that are more unethical than the exploitation of desperate patients.

Plant-based cancer cures are promoted as natural, and natural is implied to be synonymous with harmless. The marketing strategy for such products uses this fallacy and promises a cure without side effects and a treatment that avoids the often severe side effects of conventional cancer treatments. As it turns out, however, these plant-based remedies are by no means free of adverse effects. Crucially, they might interact with prescribed drugs, which could cause serious problems (Chap. 5).

By far the biggest risk of alternative cancer cures lies in the fact that they lack effectiveness. This means that cancer patients who fall for the lure of such 'natural cures' might fail to adequately treat their disease or lose valuable time to treat it effectively. This is a form of (often self-imposed) medical neglect which almost inevitably will end in tragedy.

3.2   Homeopathy

Homeopathy was invented by the German physician, Samuel Hahnemann (1755–1843). In Hahnemann's time, conventional treatments were often more dangerous than the disease they were supposed to cure. Consequently, Hahnemann's relatively harmless treatments with highly diluted substances were an almost instant, worldwide success.[35]

Many consumers confuse homeopathy with herbal medicine; yet the two are fundamentally different. Herbal medicines (Sect. 3.1) are plant extracts full of potentially active ingredients. Homeopathic remedies can be based on any material, and there are thousands of different ones on the market.

Homeopathic remedies are typically so dilute that they contain not a single molecule of the substance advertised on the bottle. The most frequently used dilution (homeopaths call them 'potencies') is a 'C30'. A C30-potency has been diluted 30 times at a ratio of 1:100 (Fig. 3.3). This means that one drop of the starting material is dissolved in 1,000,000,000,000,000,000,000,000,000,000,000,000,000,000,000,000,000,

---

[35] https://www.hive.co.uk/Product/Professor-Edzard-Ernst/Homeopathy---The-Undiluted-Facts--Including-a-Comprehensive-A-Z-Lexicon/19719982.

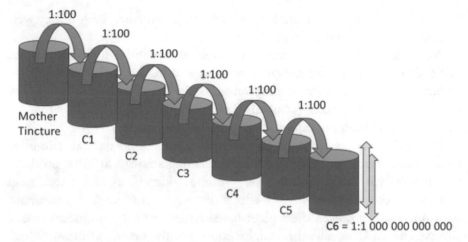

Fig. 3.3 The production of a homeopathic remedy. The starting material, called mother tincture, is diluted 1:100 and shaken (yellow arrows) to generate a C1 potency. This is again diluted and shaken to give a C2 potency, etc., etc. After 12 such dilution steps, the chances that the remedy contains a single molecule of the mother tincture are zero. Homeopaths nevertheless claim that this unique process of making a homeopathic remedy makes it not weaker but stronger with every dilution step [Copyright E Ernst]

000,000,000 drops of diluent (usually a water/alcohol mixture)—and that roughly equates to less than one molecule of the original substance per all the molecules of the universe.

Homeopaths claim that their remedies work via some undefined form of 'energy' or 'vital force' and that the manufacturing process transfers this 'energy' or information from one to the next dilution. They also believe that the process of diluting and shaking their remedies, which they call potentisation, renders them not less but more potent.

Homeopathic remedies are usually prescribed according to the 'like cures like' principle: if, for instance, a patient suffers from runny eyes, a homeopath might prescribe a remedy made of onion, because an onion can make our eyes water; and if she suffers from insomnia, a homeopath might prescribe coffea C30, because coffee keeps us awake.

The assumptions of homeopathy contradict the known laws of nature. In other words, we do not fail to comprehend how homeopathy works, as many homeopaths like to claim, but we understand that it cannot work unless the known laws of nature are wrong.

Today, around 500 clinical trials of homeopathy have been published. We can therefore expect that about 100 of them yield positive results by chance alone. It is those studies that homeopaths tend to quote in their attempts to convince the public that homeopathy is effective. However, the totality of this reliable evidence fails to show that homeopathic remedies are more than placebos.[36]

Numerous official statements from various countries confirm the absurdity and ineffectiveness of homeopathy, for instance:

- "The principles of homeopathy contradict known chemical, physical and biological laws and persuasive scientific trials proving its effectiveness are not available" (Russian Academy of Sciences, Russia)
- "Homeopathy should not be used to treat health conditions that are chronic, serious, or could become serious. People who choose homeopathy may put their health at risk if they reject or delay treatments for which there is good evidence for safety and effectiveness." (National Health and Medical Research Council, Australia)
- "Homeopathic remedies don't meet the criteria of evidence-based medicine." (Hungarian Academy of Sciences, Hungary)
- "The incorporation of anthroposophical and homeopathic products in the Swedish directive on medicinal products would run counter to several of the fundamental principles regarding medicinal products and evidence-based medicine." (Swedish Academy of Sciences, Sweden)
- "There is no good-quality evidence that homeopathy is effective as a treatment for any health condition" (National Health Service, England)

Despite this overwhelming evidence, homeopathy is being recommended by homeopaths and their professional organisations for virtually every disease, including cancer. A short excerpt of an article by THE HOMEOPATHIC COLLEGE is one example of many:

Laboratory studies in vitro and in vivo show that homeopathic drugs, in addition to having the capacity to reduce the size of tumours and to induce apoptosis, can induce protective and restorative effects. Additionally homeopathic treatment has shown effects when used as a complementary therapy for the effects of conventional cancer treatment. This confirms observations from our own clinical experience as well as that of others that when suitable remedies are selected according to individual indications as well as according to pathology and to cell-line indications and administered in the appropriate doses according to the standard principles of homeopathic posology, homeopathic treatment of cancer can be a highly effective therapy for all kinds of cancers and leukemia ...[37]

[36] Ernst E. Homeopathy: what does the "best" evidence tell us? Med J Aust. 2010 Apr 19;192(8):458–60. PMID: 20402610.

[37] http://thehomeopathiccollege.org/cancer-treatment/homeopathy-effective-cancer-treatment/.

Dr. Wurster from the 'Clinica Sta Croce' in Switzerland is even more irre-sponsible: ... *When homeopathic treatment is successful in rebuilding the immune system and reestablishing the basic regulation of the organism then tumours can disappear again. I've treated more than 1000 cancer patients homeopathically and we could even cure ... advanced and metastasizing cases...*[38]

There even are homeopathic remedies on the market specifically for curing cancer. The Vidatox website,[39] for instance, makes the following statements about their homeopathic cancer treatment:

- it is based on 5 proteins from scorpion venom;
- it is a 30C potency,
- it selectively acts on diseased cells without harming healthy ones;
- it stimulates the immune system;
- it attacks growing tumours;
- it is anti-metastatic;
- it blocks the growth of blood vessels supplying a tumour;
- it has anti-inflammatory effects;
- it has prolonged analgesic effects;
- it enhances the effects of chemo- and radiation therapies;
- it reduces the side effects of chemo- and radiation therapies;
- it is not addictive;
- it is a therapeutic alternative for human cancers;
- it is in general use in oncology;
- it has a powerful detoxification effect;
- it has no side effects;
- it improves the well-being of patients;
- its effectiveness is proven;
- the medication 'passed all the clinical trials';
- it increases survival.

With all these extraordinary claims, one would expect to find plenty of published papers on Vidatox. However, Medline offers just one article on the subject. Here is the abstract:

Complementary and alternative medicine (CAM) is the term used to describe many kinds of products, practices, and systems that are not part of conven-tional medicine. Cancer patients usually do everything they can to combat the disease, manage its symptoms, and cope with the side effects of treatment.

---

[38] https://hpathy.com/homeopathy-interviews/dr-jens-wurster/.
[39] https://cubamedicos.com/products/vidatox.

Unfortunately, patients who use CAM underestimate the risk of interaction with cancer therapy or worse they omit conventional therapy thus reducing the possibility of cancer remission. Herein we analyzed the effects of Vidatox 30 CH (venom extracted from the Junceus Rhopalurus scorpion) on hepatocellular carcinoma (HCC), the second leading cause of cancer-related deaths. We found out that Vidatox increases HCC proliferation and invasion whereas it does not seem to interact with sorafenib, the orally active multikinase inhibitor approved for the treatment of advanced hepatocellular carcinoma. Our results suggest that the concentration of Vidatox used in the present study has not anti-neoplastic effects and care must be taken in hiring Vidatox in patients with HCC.[40]

The authors of this paper also make the following comment: *There are no data from controlled clinical studies neither for Escozul nor for Vidatox 30-CH in refereed journals. The available information derived from interviews with patients involved or provided within the sites of alternative therapies. Essentially, scientific evidences about the biological activity of Vidatox in cancer cells are missing* (see Footnote 40).

But this is, of course, just one homeopathic remedy. There are thousands more. So, what does the reliable evidence tell us, is homeopathy effective in curing cancer? The scientific papers on this topic are disappointing. Many simply report test-tube experiments which tell us nothing about homeopathy's clinical value. Here is an example:

Background: Breast cancer is the second leading cause of cancer-related deaths in women. Conventional treatment such as chemotherapy, hormonal therapy and radiotherapy has decreased the mortality rate among cancer patients but has also revealed long-term side effects. Drug resistance and toxicity to normal cells compound the problems associated with the use of modern medicines. Hence, complementary or alternative treatment options are being explored. The current study, using different homeopathic potencies of Hydrastis canadensis, was conducted to distinguish between any effects they might have on hormone-dependent and independent breast cancer.

Materials and methods: The cytotoxic effect of homeopathic medicine Hydrastis on hormone-dependent (MCF 7) and hormone-independent (MDA-MB-468) breast cancer cells was assessed using viability and colony-forming assays after 48 or 72 hours of treatment. Flow cytometry-based Annexin V-PI (propidium iodide), caspase 3 and cell cycle analysis was

---

[40] Giovannini C, Baglioni M, Baron Toaldo M, Cescon M, Bolondi L, Gramantieri L. Vidatox 30 CH has tumor activating effect in hepatocellular carcinoma. Sci Rep. 2017 Mar 21;7:44685. http://doi.org/10.1038/srep44685. Erratum in: Sci Rep. 2017 Dec 22;7:46920. PMID: 28322221; PMCID: PMC5359575.

performed following treatment of cells with mother tincture or various potencies of Hydrastis (1C, 2C, 30C, 200C).

Results: Different potencies of Hydrastis displayed selective cytotoxic effects against MCF 7 cells, but only marginal effects against MDA-MB-468. The maximum cytotoxicity was established in the case of 1C following 72 h of treatment. Treatment of breast cancer cells revealed an increase in the G0/G1 cell population, along with an increase in the caspase 3 levels and induction of apoptosis.

Conclusion: Hydrastis may have a selective cytotoxic effect against hormone-dependent breast cancer MCF 7 cells, leading to cell cycle arrest in the G0/G1 phase, which could be the plausible reason for the induction of apoptosis. The results need to be validated in vivo.[41]

And here is the abstract of an equally misleading article entitled 'How homeopathic medicine works in cancer treatment':

In the current scenario of medical sciences, homeopathy, the most popular system of therapy, is recognized as one of the components of complementary and alternative medicine (CAM) across the world. Despite, a long debate is continuing whether homeopathy is just a placebo or more than it, homeopathy has been considered to be safe and cost-effectiveness therapeutic modality. A number of human ailments ranging from common to serious have been treated with homeopathy. However, selection of appropriate medicines against a disease is cumbersome task as total spectrum of symptoms of a patient guides this process. Available data suggest that homeopathy has potency not only to treat various types of cancers but also to reduce the side effects caused by standard therapeutic modalities like chemotherapy, radiotherapy or surgery. Although homeopathy has been widely used for management of cancers, its efficacy is still under question. In the present review, the anti-cancer effect of various homeopathic drugs against different kinds of cancers has been discussed and future course of action has also been suggested.[42]

Other investigations use animal models which are not necessarily applicable to human cancer patients:

Ultra low doses used in homeopathic medicines are reported to have healing potential for various diseases but their action remains controversial. In this

---

[41] Khan S, Nayak D, Khurana A, Manchanda RK, Tandon C, Tandon S. In Vitro Assessment of Homeopathic Potencies of Hydrastis canadensis on Hormone-Dependent and Independent Breast Cancer. Homeopathy. 2020 July 1. http://doi.org/10.1055/s-0040-1709668. Epub ahead of print. PMID: 32610349.

[42] Yadav R, Jee B, Rao KS. How homeopathic medicine works in cancer treatment: deep insight from clinical to experimental studies. J Exp Ther Oncol. 2019 Jan;13(1):71–76. PMID: 30658031.

study we have investigated the antitumour and antimetastatic activity of selected homeopathic medicines against transplanted tumours in mice. It was found that Ruta graveolens 200c and Hydrastis canadensis 200c significantly increased the lifespan of Ehrlich Ascites Carcinoma and Dalton's Lymphoma Ascites induced tumour-bearing animals by 49.7%, and 69.4% respectively. Moreover there was 95.6% and 95.8% reduction of solid tumour volume in Ruta 200c and Hydrastis 200c treated animals on the 31st day after tumour inoculation. Hydrastis 1M given orally significantly inhibited the growth of developed solid tumours produced by DLA cells and increased the lifespan of tumour bearing animals. Some 9 out of 15 animals with developed tumours were completely tumour free after treatment with Hydrastis 1M. Significant anti-metastatic activity was also found in B16F-10 melanoma-bearing animals treated with Thuja1M, Hydrastis 1M and Lycopodium1M. This was evident from the inhibition of lung tumour nodule formation, morphological and histopathological analysis of lung and decreased levels of gamma-GT in serum, a cellular marker of proliferation. These findings support that homeopathic preparations of Ruta and Hydrastis have significant antitumour activity. The mechanism of action of these medicines is not known at present.[43]

Proper clinical studies are far and few between. In one such investigation, data were collected retrospectively from cancer patients who had undergone homeopathic treatment complementary to conventional anti-cancer treatment at the Medical University of Vienna, Austria. A total of 54 cancer patients fulfilled the inclusion criteria. They suffered from different types of cancer: glioblastoma, lung, cholangiocellular and pancreatic carcinomas, metastasized sarcoma, and renal cell carcinoma. Median overall survival was compared to expert expectations of survival outcomes by specific cancer type and was significantly prolonged across all cancers. The authors concluded that *extended survival time in this sample of cancer patients with fatal prognosis but additive homeopathic treatment is interesting. However, findings are based on a small sample, and with only limited data available about patient and treatment characteristics. The relationship between homeopathic treatment and survival time requires prospective investigation in larger samples possibly using matched-pair control analysis or randomized trials.*[44]

[43] Es S, Kuttan G, Kc P, Kuttan R. Effect of homeopathic medicines on transplanted tumors in mice. Asian Pac J Cancer Prev. 2007 July–Sept;8(3):390–4. PMID: 18159975.

[44] Gaertner K, Müllner M, Friehs H, Schuster E, Marosi C, Muchitsch I, Frass M, Kaye AD. Additive homeopathy in cancer patients: Retrospective survival data from a homeopathic outpatient unit at the Medical University of Vienna. Complement Ther Med. 2014 Apr;22(2):320–32. http://doi.org/10.1016/j.ctim.2013.12.014. Epub 2014 Jan 8. PMID: 24731904.

As the authors correctly noted, due to a range of serious weaknesses,[45] such studies tell us little about any causal effects.

But are there no prospective clinical trials? I know of just one such investigation. The aim of this study which (published also by the above-mentioned Viennese researcher) was to investigate whether additive homeopathy might influence quality of life (QoL) and survival in non-small cell lung cancer (NSCLC) patients. In this prospective, randomized, placebo-controlled, double-blind, three-arm, multi-centre, phase III study, the researchers evaluated the possible effects of additive homeopathic treatment compared to placebo in patients with stage IV NSCLC, with respect to QoL in the two randomized groups and survival time in all three groups. In total, 150 patients with stage IV NSCLC were included in the study:

- 51 patients received individualized homeopathic remedies plus conventional treatments,
- 47 received placebo plus conventional treatments,
- 52 control patients without any homeopathic treatment were treated with conventional therapies and observed for survival only.

The results showed that QoL as well as functional and symptom scales showed significant improvement in the homeopathy group when compared with placebo after 9 and 18 weeks of homeopathic treatment. Median survival time was significantly longer in the homeopathy group (435 days) versus placebo (257 days) as well as versus control (228 days). Survival rate in the homeopathy group differed significantly from placebo and from control. The authors concluded that *QoL improved significantly in the homeopathy group compared with placebo. In addition, survival was significantly longer in the homeopathy group versus placebo and control. A higher QoL might have contributed to the prolonged survival. The study suggests that homeopathy positively influences not only QoL but also survival.*[46]

While these results seem encouraging, there are numerous concerns about this study. Firstly, the article has no methods section (the abstract is followed

---

[45] Aust N. Prolonged lifetime by adjunct homeopathy in cancer patients-A case of immortal time bias. Complement Ther Med. 2016 Feb;24:80. http://doi.org/10.1016/j.ctim.2015.12.011. Epub 2015 Dec 30. PMID: 26860806.

[46] Frass M, Lechleitner P, Gründling C, Pirker C, Grasmuk-Siegl E, Domayer J, Hochmair M, Gaertner K, Duscheck C, Muchitsch I, Marosi C, Schumacher M, Zöchbauer-Müller S, Manchanda RK, Schrott A, Burghuber O. Homeopathic Treatment as an Add-On Therapy May Improve Quality of Life and Prolong Survival in Patients with Non-Small Cell Lung Cancer: A Prospective, Randomized, Placebo-Controlled, Double-Blind, Three-Arm, Multicenter Study. Oncologist. 2020 Oct 3. http://doi.org/10.1002/onco.13548. Epub ahead of print. PMID: 33010094.

by several tables and a discussion), and the reader is left guessing much of the methodological details. Secondly, the paper raises several questions:

- What is the purpose of group 3? The authors call it a control group and state it allows assessing the real homeopathic effect on the homeopathic cohort as the real effect will be the natural historical effect minus the placebo effect and the homeopathic effect. However, this does not make much sense.
- The study seems under-powered, i.e. it was too small to allow definitive and generalizable conclusions.
- The paper does not disclose the full list of conventional treatments the patients received, and whether they differed between the 3 groups.
- The study used individualised homeopathy according to Hahnemann's instructions. Yet, Hahnemann's instructions also strictly forbid combining his approach with other types of treatment.

The first author of this trial has published many studies of homeopathy for several different conditions. Their results are invariably positive. Perhaps this should make us wary (in fact, the study is currently under investigation for irregularities). In any case, this study requires independent replications.

Until there is reliable evidence, we cannot categorise homeopathy as an effective treatment for cancer. On the contrary, We ought to warn patients not to use homeopathy as a replacement of effective therapies. Doing so would almost certainly reduce the chances of survival.

Plausibility	👎
Effectiveness	👎
Safety	👍
Cost	👍
Risk/benefit balance	👎

3.3   Diets

Consumers' interest in diets is keen. According to a 2020 survey, veganism was the most frequently searched diet type followed by vegetarianism, keto-genic diet, and low-carbohydrate diet.[47] Cancer patients are particularly interested in diet, not least because they are bombarded with claims that this or that modification of their eating habits would cure their cancer. A 2019 survey of Canadian naturopath,[48] for instance, showed that the top 5 nutritional recommendations for children with cancer were:

- anti-inflammatory diets (77.9%),
- dairy restriction (66.2%),
- Mediterranean diet (66.2%),
- gluten restriction (61.8%),
- ketogenic diet (57.4%).

The number, nature and names of diets promoted as cancer cures are bewildering. Here is but a small selection:

- Anthroposophical diet,
- Alkaline diet,
- Beetroot diet according to Seeger,
- Breuss cancer cure,
- Budwig diet,
- Evers diet,
- Fasting according to Buchinger,
- Hay's diet,
- Henderson diet,
- Kelly diet,
- Kousmine diet,
- Makrobiotic diet,
- Mayr diet,
- Moerman diet,
- Schnitzer diet,

[47] Kamiński M, Skonieczna-Żydecka K, Nowak JK, Stachowska E. Global and local diet popu-larity rankings, their secular trends, and seasonal variation in Google Trends data. Nutrition. 2020 Feb 12;79–80:110759. http://doi.org/10.1016/j.nut.2020.110759. Epub ahead of print. PMID: 32563767.

[48] Psihogios A, Ennis JK, Seely D. Naturopathic Oncology Care for Pediatric Cancers: A Practice Survey. Integr Cancer Ther. 2019 Jan–Dec;18:1534735419878504. http://doi.org/10.1177/153473 5419878504. PMID: 31566009; PMCID: PMC6769230.

- Schrot diet,
- Waerland diet,
- Young diet.

There is no doubt that an unhealthy diet can be a risk factor for developing cancer. Thus diet can be important in the prevention of cancer (Chap. 2).[49] Proponents of SCAM, however, tend to go further and claim that following a certain diet will cure the cancer or at least impede its progress. Yet, our 1996 review of the evidence found no convincing data to support these hypotheses.[50] In the following section, I will focus on a few examples of the most popular diets and discuss whether any new evidence has since emerged.

Alkaline Diet

The 'Alkaline Diet' is based on the assumption that some foods make our body acid which is alleged to be bad for our general health causing a range of diseases, including cancer. This website[51] (one of thousands on the subject) is an example for the level of misinformation that is currently out there:

> When a food is ingested, digested, and absorbed, each component of that food will present itself to the kidneys as either an acid-forming compound or a base-forming one. And when the sum total of all the acid-producing and the base-producing micro and macronutrients are tabulated, we're left with a calculated acid-base load.
>
> One common problem with most industrialized societies is that our diets produce what's called a "low grade chronic metabolic acidosis." This means we're in a chronic state of high acidity. Since the body must, at all costs, operate at a stable pH, any dietary acid load ha to be neutralized by one of a number of homeostatic base-producing mechanisms. Although the pH of the body is maintained, many cells of the body will suffer.
>
> A cancerous cell is acidic. If your body is in a constant state of over-acidification, it becomes impossible for healthy cells to regenerate. Cancer cells thrive in an overly acidic environment. By taking action to become more alkaline, you can make it more difficult for cancer cells to regenerate.

---

[49] Rinninella E, Mele MC, Cintoni M, Raoul P, Ianiro G, Salerno L, Pozzo C, Bria E, Muscaritoli M, Molfino A, Gasbarrini A. The Facts about Food after Cancer Diagnosis: A Systematic Review of Prospective Cohort Studies. Nutrients. 2020 Aug 5;12(8):2345. http://doi.org/10.3390/nu12082345. PMID: 32764484; PMCID: PMC7468771.

[50] Ernst E, Cassileth B. Cancer diets, fads and facts. Cancer Prevent Int 1996; 2: 181–187.

[51] https://www.acidalkalinediet.net/anti-cancer-diet.php.

Eating an acid/alkaline balanced diet is the key to staying healthy. Understanding the pH of the foods that you eat is relative to the state of your body's health.

The goal of the acid alkaline balance diet, also known as the alkaline diet and the alkaline ash diet, is to achieve an optimal balance between acid-forming and alkaline-forming foods. The anti cancer diet greatly reduces the strain on the body's acid-detoxification systems.

Despite a plethora of claims to the contrary, the assumption that the alkaline diet can treat cancer lacks evidential support. A systematic review concluded *that despite the promotion of the alkaline diet and alkaline water by the media and salespeople, there is almost no actual research to either support or disprove these ideas. This systematic review of the literature revealed a lack of evidence for or against diet acid load and/or alkaline water for the initiation or treatment of cancer. Promotion of alkaline diet and alkaline water to the public for cancer prevention or treatment is not justified.*[52]

The food intake has hardly any influence on the tightly regulated acidity of the blood of a healthy individual. If a patient's blood pH (a measure of acidity) would ever go outside its narrow range of 7.35 and 7.45, she would be seriously ill and require intensive care to save her life. Yet, proponents of the Alkaline diet claim that the bodies of many people are too acidic and that this surplus on acidity causes or promotes cancer. These claims are demonstrably false. Proponents furthermore assume that certain foods, like dairy products or meat, render our bodies acid. This is notion also not true. The Alkaline diet is at best useless, at worse it can cause harm through malnutrition.

Plausibility	👎
Effectiveness	👎
Safety	👎
Cost	👍
Risk/benefit balance	👎

---

[52] Fenton TR, Huang T. Systematic review of the association between dietary acid load, alkaline water and cancer. BMJ Open. 2016 June 13;6(6):e010438. http://doi.org/10.1136/bmjopen-2015-010438. PMID: 27297008; PMCID: PMC4916623.

Anthroposophical Diet

The anthroposophic diet[53] is essentially a vegetarian diet based on the principles of Rudolf Steiner's anthroposophic medicine (Sect. 3.2). Dairy products and eggs are permitted, while the consumption of meat, fish, soy and industrially processed foods such as sugar and white flour should be restricted. As Steiner felt that each individual's choice of food should be respected, this diet is not strict but consists of mere recommendations and guidelines.

Anthroposophic nutritional theory divides plants into

- root vegetables,
- vegetables from leaves and stems,
- fruit and blossom.

According to anthroposophic belief, the effects of these nutrients on health differ, e.g.:

- root vegetables have positive effects on nerves and the head,
- leafy vegetables, salads and cabbage strengthen heart and lungs,
- fruits and seeds stimulate digestion and metabolism.

In order to achieve an optimal balance, food from all three categories should be eaten daily. None of these assumptions are based on facts. Since biodynamic cultivation is another invention of Rudolf Steiner, it does not surprise that followers of anthroposophic nutrition are told to consume fresh and unprocessed foods grown biodynamically.

Even though it is recommended as a cancer cure, there is no evidence that the anthroposophic diet affects the natural history of any type of cancer.

Plausibility	👎
Effectiveness	👎
Safety	👍
Cost	👍
Risk/benefit balance	👎

---

[53] https://dr-barbara-hendel.com/en/nutrition/forms-of-nutrition/anthroposophical-diet/.

Breuss Cancer Cure

The Breuss cancer cure (BCC) is a diet of fruits and vegetables taken in liquid form for a period of 42 days. It is claimed to starve the cancer cells by not providing solid food proteins, while not harming normal cells. The erroneous assumption is that cancer cells can only live on the protein of solid food.

It seems fairly obvious that calorie restriction would slow the growth of a cancer; however, for obvious reasons, it cannot last for prolonged periods. As soon as the calorie supply is reinstated, the cancer growth can be expected to resume. Therefore the assumptions of the BCC lack biological plausibility.

The BCC is based on the Breuss vegetable juice that consists of:

- 55% red beet root,
- 20% carrots,
- 20% celery root,
- 3% raw potato,
- 2% radishes.

There is no evidence to support any of the claims made for the BCC. As conventional cancer treatments are not allowed with this regimen, and as the diet carries the risk of malnutrition, the BCC even seems outright dangerous.

Plausibility	👎
Effectiveness	👎
Safety	👎
Cost	👍
Risk/benefit balance	👎

Budwig Diet

The Budwig diet is based on flaxseed oil, cottage cheese and fruit juice. The diet is named after its creator, the pharmacist Johanna Budwig, who assumed that a diet high in polyunsaturated fatty acids would energize healthy cells to keep cancer from spreading. Patients are encouraged to spend time exposing their skin to the sun to promote vitamin D production.

The Budwig diet avoids foods that are claimed to prevent the body from functioning at its optimal level. Forbidden are thus all processed foods and other ingredients deemed to be unhealthy, including:

- meats that contain antibiotics or artificial hormones,
- shellfish,
- hydrogenated oils and trans fats,
- soy products,
- white sugar,
- animal fats,
- refined grains,
- foods containing artificial preservatives.

Budwig's assumptions lack plausibility. There is no evidence that her diet has any effects on the natural history of any cancer.

Plausibility	👎
Effectiveness	👎
Safety	👍
Cost	👍
Risk/benefit balance	👎

Gerson Diet

The Gerson diet was developed about 100 years ago by the German doctor Max Gerson (1881–1959). He was convinced that the diet, which was originally developed as a treatment for tuberculosis, had cured his migraines. Subsequently, it was promoted for a range of illnesses. The 'Gerson Institute' states that "*Over the past 60 years, thousands of people have used the Gerson Therapy to recover from a variety of illnesses, including: Cancer (including melanoma, breast cancer, prostate cancer, colon cancer, lymphoma and more)…*".[54]

The Gerson diet is essentially a starvation diet; it consists of ingesting raw and organically-grown vegetables and freshly-pressed vegetable juices

---

[54] https://gerson.org/gerpress/.

(up to 13 large glasses/day). In addition, regular coffee enemas are administered allegedly stimulating the liver to detoxify the body and a range of supplements is usually prescribed. The treatment is normally administered in specialised hospitals, and the costs for the whole treatment package are high.

There is no good evidence that the Gerson therapy is effective as a cancer cure. The only controlled clinical trial of a Gerson-like diet for cancer generated a negative result; here is its abstract[55]:

Conventional medicine has had little to offer patients with inoperable pancreatic adenocarcinoma; thus, many patients seek alternative treatments. The National Cancer Institute, in 1998, sponsored a randomized, phase III, controlled trial of proteolytic enzyme therapy versus chemotherapy. Because most eligible patients refused random assignment, the trial was changed in 2001 to a controlled, observational study.

METHODS

All patients were seen by one of the investigators at Columbia University, and patients who received enzyme therapy were seen by the participating alternative practitioner. Of 55 patients who had inoperable pancreatic cancer, 23 elected gemcitabine-based chemotherapy, and 32 elected enzyme treatment, which included pancreatic enzymes, nutritional supplements, detoxification, and an organic diet. Primary and secondary outcomes were overall survival and quality of life, respectively.

RESULTS

At enrollment, the treatment groups had no statistically significant differences in patient characteristics, pathology, quality of life, or clinically meaningful laboratory values. Kaplan-Meier analysis found a 9.7-month difference in median survival between the chemotherapy group (median survival, 14 months) and enzyme treatment groups (median survival, 4.3 months) and found an adjusted-mortality hazard ratio of the enzyme group compared with the chemotherapy group of 6.96 ($P < 0.001$). At 1 year, 56% of chemotherapy group patients were alive, and 16% of enzyme-therapy patients were alive. The quality of life ratings was better in the chemotherapy group than in the enzyme-treated group ($P < 0.01$).

CONCLUSION

Among patients who have pancreatic cancer, those who chose gemcitabine-based chemotherapy survived more than three times as long (14.0 v 4.3 months) and had better quality of life than those who chose proteolytic enzyme treatment.

---

[55] Chabot JA, Tsai WY, Fine RL, Chen C, Kumah CK, Antman KA, Grann VR. Pancreatic proteolytic enzyme therapy compared with gemcitabine-based chemotherapy for the treatment of pancreatic cancer. J Clin Oncol. 2010 Apr 20;28(12):2058–63. http://doi.org/10.1200/JCO.2009.22.8429. Epub 2009 Aug 17. PMID: 19687327; PMCID: PMC2860407.

A recent review stated that *no conclusions about the effectiveness of the Gerson therapy, either as an adjuvant to other cancer therapies or as a cure, can be drawn.*[56]

The Gerson diet deprives cancer patients of vital nutrients; in addition, it can drastically impair their quality of life. Most patients find it very hard to follow, and the many who fail to adhere to it are then told that it is their fault, if their cancer does not respond. Thus, they would die not merely deprived of their funds and quality of life but also feeling guilty.

Plausibility	👎
Effectiveness	👎
Safety	👎
Cost	👎
Risk/benefit balance	👎

Ketogenic Diet

The Ketogenic diet (KD) is low in glucose and thus claimed to be capable of starving cancer cells to death and thus restricting tumour growth.

Two systematic reviews of the KD as a treatment of cancer are available:

- The efficacy and benefits of ketogenic diets (KD) have recently been gaining worldwide and remain a controversial topic in oncology. This systematic review therefore presents and evaluates the clinical evidence on isocaloric KD dietary regimes and reveals that evidence supporting the effects of isocaloric ketogenic dietary regimes on tumour development and progression as well as reduction in side effects of cancer therapy is missing. Furthermore, an array of potential side effects should be carefully considered before applying KD to cancer patients. In regard to counselling cancer patients considering a KD, more robust and consistent clinical evidence

---

[56] Gerson Therapy (PDQ®) Health Professional Version, PDQ Integrative, Alternative, and Complementary Therapies Editorial Board. Published online: April 11, 2016. https://www.ncbi.nlm.nih.gov/books/NBK66029/.

is necessary before the KD can be recommended for any single cancer diagnosis or as an adjunct therapy.[57]

- Although most preclinical studies indicate a therapeutic potential for ketogenic diets in cancer treatment, it is now becoming clear that not all tumours might respond positively. Early clinical trials have investigated ketogenic diets as a monotherapy and—while showing the safety of the approach even in advanced cancer patients—largely failed to prove survival prolonging effects. However, it gradually became clear that the greatest potential for ketogenic diets is as adjuvant treatments combined with pro-oxidative or targeted therapies initiated in early stages of the disease. Beneficial effects on body composition and quality of life have also been found. Summary: Ketogenic diets against cancer are worth further exploration, both in the laboratory and clinically. Patients wishing to undertake a ketogenic diet during therapy should receive dietary counselling to avoid common mistakes and optimize compliance. Future research should focus more on important clinical endpoints.[58]

The cautiously positive verdict of the second review seems surprising and unjustified, as it is based on only one single RCT to support it. This study compared a diet of 70% fat, 25% protein, and 5% carbohydrate to the dietary recommendations of the American Cancer Society over 12 weeks in women with ovarian or endometrial cancer. About 25% of the women had concurrent chemotherapy. Women in the ketogenic diet group, but not the American Cancer Society diet group, experienced a significant increase in physical functioning. Among women receiving no chemotherapy, energy levels also increased significantly in the ketogenic diet group only. After 12 weeks, the ketogenic diet group reported more cravings for salty foods, but less frequent cravings for starchy foods and fast food fats, which was significantly different from the control group after adjusting for baseline values and chemotherapy status. The ketogenic diet reduced insulin levels as well as total, android and visceral fat mass to a significantly greater extent than the American Cancer Society diet, while total lean mass remained constant

[57] Erickson N, Boscheri A, Linke B, Huebner J. Systematic review: isocaloric ketogenic dietary regimes for cancer patients. Med Oncol. 2017 May;34(5):72. http://doi.org/10.1007/s12032-017-0930-5. Epub 2017 Mar 28. PMID: 28353094.

[58] Klement RJ. The emerging role of ketogenic diets in cancer treatment. Curr Opin Clin Nutr Metab Care. 2019 Mar;22(2):129–134. http://doi.org/10.1097/MCO.0000000000000540. PMID: 30531479.

in both groups. Adherence was estimated at about 80% in both groups, and again the ketogenic diet did not show serious side effects.[59] [60]

This study did not include clinical endpoints relevant to cancer progression. Thus, there is no reliable evidence to show that the KD affects the natural history of any cancer.

Plausibility	👎
Effectiveness	👎
Safety	👍
Cost	👍
Risk/benefit balance	👎

Macrobiotic Diet

The macrobiotic diet was popularized in the 1930s by George Ohsawa (1893–1966) who claimed to have cured his tuberculosis with it. Michio Kushi (1916–2014) further popularised macrobiotics during the 1950s.

The diet is based mainly on locally grown whole grain cereals, pulses, vegetables, seaweed, fermented soy products and fruit. Nightshade vegetables (e.g. tomatoes, peppers, potatoes, eggplant), spinach, beets and avocados are used sparingly or not at all. The principle is that yin foods must be in balance with yang foods, an assumption that harps back to Traditional Chinese Medicine but lacks plausibility.

The diet is recommended for the treatment of a very wide range of conditions, including cancer.[61] However, there is little good evidence that

---

[59] Cohen CW, Fontaine KR, Arend RC, Alvarez RD, Leath CA III, Huh WK, Bevis KS, Kim KH, Straughn JM Jr, Gower BA. A Ketogenic Diet Reduces Central Obesity and Serum Insulin in Women with Ovarian or Endometrial Cancer. J Nutr. 2018 Aug 1;148(8):1253–1260. http://doi.org/10.1093/jn/nxy119. PMID: 30137481.

[60] Cohen CW, Fontaine KR, Arend RC, Soleymani T, Gower BA. Favorable Effects of a Ketogenic Diet on Physical Function, Perceived Energy, and Food Cravings in Women with Ovarian or Endometrial Cancer: A Randomized, Controlled Trial. Nutrients. 2018 Aug 30;10(9):1187. http://doi.org/10.3390/nu10091187. PMID: 30200193; PMCID: PMC6163837.

[61] Kushi LH, Cunningham JE, Hebert JR, Lerman RH, Bandera EV, Teas J. The macrobiotic diet in cancer. J Nutr. 2001 Nov;131(11 Suppl):3056S–64S. http://doi.org/10.1093/jn/131.11.3056S. PMID: 11694648.

following a macrobiotic diet affects the natural history of any form of cancer.[62][63]

Rigorous adherence to a macrobiotic diet can cause severe nutritional deficiencies and even death. Concerns include potential delay in conventional treatment for cancer, risks associated with nutrition deficiencies, and social limitations related to the complexities of strict adherence to this diet.

Plausibility	👎
Effectiveness	👎
Safety	👎
Cost	👍
Risk/benefit balance	👎

Vegetarian and Vegan Diets

Many SCAM proponents are convinced that meat-free diets have benefits for cancer patients. The association of meat consumption and cancer risk and the role of meat-free diets in cancer prevention have been discussed in Chap. 2. The notion that vegan and vegetarian diets can cure an existing cancer is wide spread but not supported by good evidence.[64] Moreover, several investigations have shown that meat-free diets are associated with considerable health risks that are not related to cancer but nevertheless relevant. [e.g.65]

Thus there is no reliable evidence to show that vegetarian or vegan diets alter the natural history of cancer.

---

[62] Lerman RH. The macrobiotic diet in chronic disease. Nutr Clin Pract. 2010 Dec;25(6):621–6. http://doi.org/10.1177/0884533610385704. PMID: 21139126.

[63] Cunningham E, Marcason W. Is there any research to prove that a macrobiotic diet can prevent or cure cancer? J Am Diet Assoc. 2001 Sept;101(9):1030. http://doi.org/10.1016/S0002-8223(01)002 53-X. PMID: 11573754.

[64] Dinu M, Abbate R, Gensini GF, Casini A, Sofi F. Vegetarian, vegan diets and multiple health outcomes: A systematic review with meta-analysis of observational studies. Crit Rev Food Sci Nutr. 2017 Nov 22;57(17):3640–3649. http://doi.org/10.1080/10408398.2016.1138447. PMID: 26853923.

[65] Tong TYN, Appleby PN, Armstrong MEG, Fensom GK, Knuppel A, Papier K, Perez-Cornago A, Travis RC, Key TJ. Vegetarian and vegan diets and risks of total and site-specific fractures: results from the prospective EPIC-Oxford study. BMC Med. 2020 Nov 23;18(1):353. http://doi.org/10.1186/s12916-020-018 15-3. PMID: 33222682; PMCID: PMC7682057.

Plausibility	👎
Effectiveness	👎
Safety	👎
Cost	👍
Risk/benefit balance	👎

Conclusion

The collective evidence does not suggest that any of the alternative cancer diets are able to change the natural history of any form of cancer. In 2014, a German team of oncologists and scientists evaluated the following alternative cancer diets: raw vegetables and fruits, alkaline diet, macrobiotics, Gerson's regime, Budwig's and ketogenic diet. They confirmed our above-mentioned conclusions and failed to find clinical evidence supporting any of the diets. Furthermore, case reports and preclinical data pointed to the dangers of some of these diets. The authors concluded that *considering the lack of evidence of benefits from cancer diets and potential harm by malnutrition, oncologists should engage more in counselling cancer patients on such diets.*[66]

In other words, alternative cancer diets—not just the ones mentioned above, but all of them—are not supported by good evidence for effectiveness as a treatment of cancer; they have not been proven to prolong the life of cancer patients or to cure any type of cancer. In addition, they might also cause serious harm. Cancer patients should take sound nutritional advice and adopt a healthy lifestyle. But they should be wary of SCAM-practitioners suggesting an alternative dietary cure for their disease.

3.4   Non-plant-Based Supplements

The US 'National Health and Nutrition Examination Survey' (NHANES) included a total of 4575 respondents with cancer and showed that 66% of

---

[66] Huebner J, Marienfeld S, Abbenhardt C, Ulrich C, Muenstedt K, Micke O, Muecke R, Loeser C. Counseling patients on cancer diets: a review of the literature and recommendations for clinical practice. Anticancer Res. 2014 Jan;34(1):39–48. PMID: 24403443.

them reported using dietary supplements. Factors associated with the usage included:

- older age,
- white race,
- female gender,
- higher income,
- higher educational level,
- better self-reported health,
- health insurance,
- history of a previous cancer.

The survey found that the use of dietary supplements was not associated with a difference in overall survival. Dietary supplement use had increased in the past two decades among individuals with cancer, and this increase seemed to be driven mainly by an increase in the use of vitamins.[67] A similar survey showed that 74% of cancer survivors reported taking supplements. The ones that were most commonly employed were non-plant-based supplements:

- multivitamins (60%),
- calcium/vitamin D (37%),
- antioxidants (30%).[68]

Many of these non-herbal supplements are being promoted as alternative cancer cures. In this chapter, I will discuss the evidence for and against some of those that are currently popular.

Colloidal Silver

Amongst all supplements, colloidal silver occupies a special place, if only for the simple reason that it is hard to find a condition which it is not said to cure; and sadly, this includes cancer.

---

[67] Abdel-Rahman O. Dietary Supplements Use among Adults with Cancer in the United States: A Population-Based Study. Nutr Cancer. 2020 Sept 15:1–8. http://doi.org/10.1080/01635581.2020.182 0050. Epub ahead of print. PMID: 32930008.

[68] Miller P, Demark-Wahnefried W, Snyder DC, Sloane R, Morey MC, Cohen H, Kranz S, Mitchell DC, Hartman TJ. Dietary supplement use among elderly, long-term cancer survivors. J Cancer Surviv. 2008 Sept;2(3):138–48. http://doi.org/10.1007/s11764-008-0060-3. Epub 2008 July 11. PMID: 18792788; PMCID: PMC2766274.

A man claiming to sell a cure for cancer has been fined £750 following an investigation by Essex Trading Standards. Steven Cook, 54, of East Road, West Mersea, was charged with an offence under the Cancer Act after suggesting Colloidal Silver was a treatment for cancer.

Mr Cook pleaded guilty at Colchester Magistrates' Court on Friday 12 September 2015. Magistrates imposed a fine of £750 and ordered him to pay £1500 costs. Cllr Roger Hirst, Essex County Council's cabinet member for Trading Standards, said: "Trading Standards" advice to people who are considering whether to take any substance not prescribed for a medical purpose, either preventative or as a treatment, is to consult their doctor first.

"I hope the public feel safer knowing that Essex Trading Standards will take action where traders are trying to sell products which are neither medically proven nor safe."

Mr Cook runs a website, www.colloidalsilveruk.com, selling various products containing silver. One of the products on sale was "Ultimate Colloidal Silver", a liquid containing silver that Mr Cook made in his own home. Trading Standards said the website implied that the product can cure cancer—and this is an offence under the Cancer Act. Mr Cook has now updated the website and removed any claims that colloidal silver can cure some cancers.[69]

Silver is a metal that is toxic for bacteria, algae, and fungi, as it irreversibly damages enzyme systems in the cell membranes of these pathogens. Therefore, the use of silver in wound dressings, creams and coatings on medical devices used to be wide spread. The emergence of more powerful antibiotics and antiseptics have, however, rendered this all but obsolete.

Not so in SCAM! Here, colloidal silver for oral or topical use has made a renaissance—not because, but despite sound evidence. One review assessed the evidence for colloidal silver and emphasized the total lack of reliable effectiveness for any condition.[70]

Not only is colloidal silver not an effective cancer cure, but some evidence suggests that its long-term use might even cause cancer.[71] It can also result in a blue-grey discolouration of the skin known as argyria.[72] One case report

---

[69] https://www.essex.gov.uk/news.

[70] Fung MC, Bowen DL. Silver products for medical indications: risk–benefit assessment. J Toxicol Clin Toxicol. 1996;34(1):119–26. http://doi.org/10.3109/15563659609020246. PMID: 8632503.

[71] Keung YK, Wang T, Hong-Lung Hu E. Acute myeloid leukemia with complex cytogenetic abnormalities associated with long-term use of oral colloidal silver as nutritional supplement—Case report and review of literature. J Oncol Pharm Pract. 2020 Jan;26(1):212–215. http://doi.org/10.1177/107 8155219832966. Epub 2019 Mar 9. PMID: 30854923.

[72] Hadrup N, Lam HR. Oral toxicity of silver ions, silver nanoparticles and colloidal silver—a review. Regul Toxicol Pharmacol. 2014 Feb;68(1):1–7. http://doi.org/10.1016/j.yrtph.2013.11.002. Epub 2013 Nov 12. PMID: 24231525.

described a man who suffered from epilepsy after long-term colloidal silver intake, followed by a vegetative state and death.[73] An investigation from Finland concluded that *the use of quackery products such as colloidal silver can be dangerous, and their use and marketing should be controlled and restricted.*[74]

Plausibility	👎
Effectiveness	👎
Safety	👎
Cost	👍
Risk/benefit balance	👎

Enzymes

Enzyme therapy for cancer involves the administration of proteolytic enzymes by mouth. Proteolytic enzymes are large molecules that nonetheless are claimed to get absorbed in the gut. Trypsin, chymotrypsin, bromelain, papain or combinations of those enzymes are being marketed as dietary supplements and said to exert anti-cancer activities by restoring the reduced cytotoxic activity of cancer patients' blood.

Enzyme therapy has been subjected to several experimental investigations and to clinical studies in cancer patients. A systematic review claimed that enzyme therapy increases the response rates, the duration of remissions, and the overall survival times of plasmacytoma patients.[75] However, this statement is based on just one single study. Here is its abstract[76]:

[73] Mirsattari SM, Hammond RR, Sharpe MD, Leung FY, Young GB. Myoclonic status epilepticus following repeated oral ingestion of colloidal silver. Neurology. 2004 Apr 27;62(8):1408–10. http://doi.org/10.1212/01.wnl.0000120671.73335.ec. PMID: 15111684.

[74] Leino V, Airaksinen R, Viluksela M, Vähäkangas K. Toxicity of colloidal silver products and their marketing claims in Finland. Toxicol Rep. 2020 Dec 26;8:106–113. http://doi.org/10.1016/j.toxrep.2020.12.021. PMID: 33437653; PMCID: PMC7786010.

[75] Beuth J. Proteolytic enzyme therapy in evidence-based complementary oncology: fact or fiction? Integr Cancer Ther. 2008 Dec;7(4):311–6. http://doi.org/10.1177/1534735408327251. PMID: 19116226.

[76] Sakalová A, Bock PR, Dedík L, Hanisch J, Schiess W, Gazová S, Chabronová I, Holomanova D, Mistrík M, Hrubisko M. Retrolective cohort study of an additive therapy with an oral enzyme preparation in patients with multiple myeloma. Cancer Chemother Pharmacol. 2001 July;47 Suppl:S38–44. http://doi.org/10.1007/s002800170008. PMID: 11561871.

Purpose: To evaluate the impact of an additive therapy with an oral enzyme (OE) preparation given for more than 6 months additionally to standard combination chemotherapy (vincristine/melphalan/cyclophosphamide/prednisone (VMCP)- or methylprednisolone/vincristine/CCNU/cyclophosphamide/melphalan (MOCCA)-regimen) in the primary treatment of patients with multiple myeloma stages I-III.

Methods: A cohort of 265 patients with multiple myeloma stages I-III was consecutively treated at our institution in two parallel groups (control group ($n = 99$): chemotherapy +/−OE for less than 6 months; OE-group ($n = 166$): chemotherapy + OE for more than 6 months). The median follow-up time in the stages I, II, and III for the OE-group was 61, 37, and 46.5 months, respectively; for the control group the respective values were 33, 51.5, and 31.5 months. The primary endpoint of the study was disease-specific survival. Secondary endpoints were response to therapy, duration of first response and side effects. The chosen method for evaluation was the technique of a retrolective cohort analysis with a concurrent control group. Survival analysis was performed by the Kaplan-Meier method and multivariate analysis was done with the Cox proportional hazards model.

Results: Significantly higher overall response rates and longer duration of remissions were observed in the OE-group. Primary responders showed a longer mean survival time than non-responders. Additive therapy with OE given for more than 6 months decreased the hazard of death for patients at all stages of disease by approximately 60%. Observation time was not long enough to estimate the median survival for patients at stages I and II; for stage III patients it was 47 months in the control group versus 83 months for the patients treated with OE ($P = 0.0014$) which means a 3-year gain of survival time. Significant prognostic factors for survival, in the Cox regression analysis, were stage of disease and therapy with OE. The OE-therapy was generally well tolerated (3.6% of patients with mild to moderate gastrointestinal symptoms).

Conclusion: OEs represent a promising new additive therapy in multiple myeloma which will be further evaluated in a randomized phase III trial in the USA.

This study was published 20 years ago—plenty of time for an independent replication or a more rigorous clinical trial. Yet, none has so far emerged. Consequently, the evidence to suggest that enzyme therapy might be an effective treatment for any type of cancer is less than convincing.

Plausibility	👆
Effectiveness	👎

(continued)

(continued)

Safety	👍
Cost	👎
Risk/benefit balance	👎

Melatonin

Melatonin is a hormone which is secreted from the human pineal gland during night time acting as physiological regulator. In many countries, dietary supplements containing synthetically produced melatonin are commercially available. Melatonin has been suggested as a treatment of a range of conditions, including cancer.

Test-tube experiments suggest that melatonin has anti-cancer effects.[77] Its actions include the advancement of apoptosis, the arrest of the cell cycle, inhibition of metastasis, and antioxidant activity.[78] Several clinical trials of melatonin for cancer are available.

- A review of 21 clinical trials of melatonin for cancer found positive effects for complete response, partial response, and stable disease. In trials combining melatonin with chemotherapy, adjuvant melatonin therapy decreased 1-year mortality and improved outcomes of complete response, partial response, and stable disease. In these studies, melatonin also significantly reduced asthenia, leukopenia, nausea and vomiting, hypotension, and thrombocytopenia. The authors concluded that melatonin *may benefit cancer patients who are also receiving chemotherapy, radiotherapy, supportive therapy, or palliative therapy by improving survival and ameliorating the side effects of chemotherapy.*[79]

[77] Kong X, Gao R, Wang Z, Wang X, Fang Y, Gao J, Reiter RJ, Wang J. Melatonin: A Potential Therapeutic Option for Breast Cancer. Trends Endocrinol Metab. 2020 Sept 3:S1043–2760(20)30155–7. http://doi.org/10.1016/j.tem.2020.08.001. Epub ahead of print. PMID: 32893084.

[78] Samanta S. Melatonin: an endogenous miraculous indolamine, fights against cancer progression. J Cancer Res Clin Oncol. 2020 Aug;146(8):1893–1922. http://doi.org/10.1007/s00432-020-03292-w. Epub 2020 June 24. PMID: 32583237.

[79] Seely D, Wu P, Fritz H, Kennedy DA, Tsui T, Seely AJ, Mills E. Melatonin as adjuvant cancer care with and without chemotherapy: a systematic review and meta-analysis of randomized trials. Integr Cancer Ther. 2012 Dec;11(4):293–303. http://doi.org/10.1177/1534735411425484. Epub 2011 Oct 21. PMID: 22019490.

- A further systematic review of RCTs of melatonin in solid tumour cancer patients evaluated its effect on one-year survival. Ten trials were included of melatonin as either sole treatment or as adjunct treatment. Melatonin reduced the risk of death at 1 year. Effects were consistent across melatonin dose, and type of cancer. No severe adverse events were reported.[80]
- A 2012 systematic review confirmed these findings by concluding that *Melatonin as an adjuvant therapy for cancer led to substantial improvements in tumour remission, 1-year survival, and alleviation of radiochemotherapy-related side effects.*[81] Finally, a 2020 review concluded that *melatonin in combination with anticancer agents may improve the efficacy of routine medicine and survival rate of patients with cancer.*[82] Apart from its direct anticancer potential, melatonin also seems to reduce chemotherapy toxicity, while improving its therapeutic efficacy.[83]

While all this sounds encouraging, it is prudent to note several important caveats. The primary studies of melatonin suffer from significant methodological shortcomings, and their majority originate from one single Italian research group. In recent years, there have been no further clinical studies trying to replicate the initial findings. This means that definitive trials are still missing, and it would seem wise to interpret the existing evidence with caution.[84]

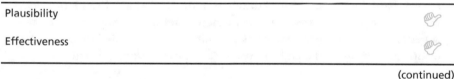

Plausibility	
Effectiveness	

(continued)

---

[80] Mills E, Wu P, Seely D, Guyatt G. Melatonin in the treatment of cancer: a systematic review of randomized controlled trials and meta-analysis. J Pineal Res. 2005 Nov;39(4):360–6. http://doi.org/10.1111/j.1600-079X.2005.00258.x. PMID: 16207291.

[81] Wang YM, Jin BZ, Ai F, Duan CH, Lu YZ, Dong TF, Fu QL. The efficacy and safety of melatonin in concurrent chemotherapy or radiotherapy for solid tumors: a meta-analysis of randomized controlled trials. Cancer Chemother Pharmacol. 2012 May;69(5):1213–20. http://doi.org/10.1007/s00280-012-1828-8. Epub 2012 Jan 24. PMID: 22271210.

[82] Pourhanifeh MH, Mehrzadi S, Kamali M, Hosseinzadeh A. Melatonin and gastrointestinal cancers: Current evidence based on underlying signaling pathways. Eur J Pharmacol. 2020 Nov 5;886:173471. http://doi.org/10.1016/j.ejphar.2020.173471. Epub 2020 Aug 30. PMID: 32877658.

[83] Iravani S, Eslami P, Dooghaie Moghadam A, Moazzami B, Mehrvar A, Hashemi MR, Mansour-Ghanaei F, Mansour-Ghanaei A, Majidzadeh-A K. The Role of Melatonin in Colorectal Cancer. J Gastrointest Cancer. 2020 Sept;51(3):748–753. http://doi.org/10.1007/s12029-019-00336-4. PMID: 31792737.

[84] Fernández-Palanca P, Méndez-Blanco C, Fondevila F, Tuñón MJ, Reiter RJ, Mauriz JL, González-Gallego J. Melatonin as an Antitumor Agent against Liver Cancer: An Updated Systematic Review. Antioxidants (Basel). 2021 Jan 12;10(1):E103. http://doi.org/10.3390/antiox10010103. PMID: 33445767.

(continued)

Safety	👍
Cost	👍
Risk/benefit balance	🤚

Probiotics

Probiotics consist of microorganisms claimed to convey health benefits by improving or restoring the gut flora. Their current use goes back to Nobel laureate Élie Metchnikoff, who believed that yoghurt consumption prolongs life, a claim which was later even supported by some population studies.[85]

Probiotics are promoted for many diseases, including cancer. This quote, for instance, is from a publication specialising in (mis)informing the public about SCAM:

> Colon cancer could be reversed just with probiotics that change the gut's bacteria—and the disease can be prevented in the first place by eating whole grains, such as brown rice and whole-wheat bread, every day, two new research studies have found. In a breakthrough study that could herald in a new drugs-free approach to treating colon cancer, researchers have discovered that sufferers lack certain enzymes known as metabolites, simple 'building-block' compounds, in their gut, and this can cause inflammation and cancer...[86]

Imbalances in the gut microbiota might contribute to the progress of certain cancers. Several therapeutic methods are available to remedy the problem, such as the administration of prebiotics (compounds that induce the growth or activity of the gut microbiome) or probiotics, as well as microbiota transplantation via faecal transplants.

---

[85] Schmid D, Song M, Zhang X, Willett WC, Vaidya R, Giovannucci EL, Michels KB. Yogurt consumption in relation to mortality from cardiovascular disease, cancer, and all causes: a prospective investigation in 2 cohorts of US women and men. Am J Clin Nutr. 2020 Mar 1;111(3):689–697. http://doi.org/10.1093/ajcn/nqz345. PMID: 31968071; PMCID: PMC7049530.

[86] https://www.wddty.com/news/2017/09/probiotics-could-reverse-colon-cancer.html?utm_source=Boomtrain&utm_medium=email&utm_campaign=enews_18092017&bt_ee=euUX7yQ7OOO6CU1n/e8H9k2OyIDolp+9Le03xGsYlQkq3y0NGSOt/xoJRRS2SCia&bt_ts=1505736085686.

While there is some preliminary evidence to suggest that probiotics might reduce the risk of certain cancers (Chap. 2), there is no good evidence to show that they cure any type of cancer.[87]

Plausibility	
Effectiveness	
Safety	
Cost	
Risk/benefit balance	

Shark Cartilage

Shark cartilage products are made from the dried skeletons of sharks. Numerous supplements are being promoted as cancer cures, and the annual world market for such products exceeds US $30 million. The naïve assumption is that sharks do not get cancer; thus, their cartilage must be a cancer cure.[88] This notion is wrong on two accounts: firstly, sharks do get cancer; and secondly is their skeleton not a cure for cancer.

Two glycoproteins (sphyrnastatin 1 and 2) have been isolated from the cartilage of the hammerhead shark and were reported to exhibit antiangiogenic activity inhibiting blood supply, an effect which could theoretically be useful as a cancer therapy.[89] Other mechanisms of action have also been suggested: shark cartilage is claimed to kill cancer cells directly, and it is said to stimulate the immune system. Due to the large size of the molecules, it is questionable whether, after oral administration, the sphyrnastatins ever reach the bloodstream in sufficiently high concentrations.

[87] Khani S, Hosseini HM, Taheri M, Nourani MR, Imani Fooladi AA. Probiotics as an alternative strategy for prevention and treatment of human diseases: a review. Inflamm Allergy Drug Targets. 2012 Apr;11(2):79–89. http://doi.org/10.2174/187152812800392832. PMID: 22280243.

[88] Ostrander GK, Cheng KC, Wolf JC, Wolfe MJ. Shark cartilage, cancer and the growing threat of pseudoscience. Cancer Res. 2004 Dec 1;64(23):8485–91. http://doi.org/10.1158/0008-5472.CAN-04-2260. Erratum in: Cancer Res. 2005 Jan 1;65(1):374. PMID: 15574750.

[89] Rabbani-Chadegani A, Abdossamadi S, Bargahi A, Yousef-Masboogh M. Identification of low-molecular-weight protein (SCP1) from shark cartilage with anti-angiogenesis activity and sequence similarity to parvalbumin. J Pharm Biomed Anal. 2008 Feb 13;46(3):563–7. http://doi.org/10.1016/j.jpba.2007.10.029. Epub 2007 Nov 1. PMID: 18093782.

The only placebo-controlled RCT of cartilage as cancer treatment published in a peer-reviewed scientific journal compared shark cartilage to placebo in addition to standard care. In 83 patients having either advanced breast or advanced colon cancer, there was no difference in the quality of life or survival rate between the two groups. The authors concluded that *this trial was unable to demonstrate any suggestion of efficacy for this shark cartilage product in patients with advanced cancer.*[90] A review of the evidence stated that the promotion of crude shark cartilage extracts as a cure for cancer has contributed to at least two significant negative outcomes: *a dramatic decline in shark populations and a diversion of patients from effective cancer treatments... The fact that people think shark cartilage consumption can cure cancer illustrates the serious potential impacts of pseudoscience* (see Footnote 84).

Thus shark cartilage supplements are proven to kill sharks but not cancer.

Plausibility	👎
Effectiveness	👎
Safety	👍
Cost	👎
Risk/benefit balance	👎

Vitamin C

In 1747, James Lind conducted the first documented controlled clinical trial in the history of medicine. He treated a small group of healthy sailors with a range of different remedies to see whether one of these regimens might be effective in preventing scurvy. The results showed that lemon and lime juice—effectively vitamin C—was indeed effective. Of course, Lind did not know that the effective principle in his lemon/lime juice was vitamin C. The Hungarian physiologist Albert Szent-Gyorgyi (1893–1986) discovered vitamin C (ascorbic acid) only ~200 years later (and received the Nobel Prize for it in 1937).

---

[90] Loprinzi CL, Levitt R, Barton DL, Sloan JA, Atherton PJ, Smith DJ, Dakhil SR, Moore DF Jr, Krook JE, Rowland KM Jr, Mazurczak MA, Berg AR, Kim GP; North Central Cancer Treatment Group. Evaluation of shark cartilage in patients with advanced cancer: a North Central Cancer Treatment Group trial. Cancer. 2005 July 1;104(1):176–82. http://doi.org/10.1002/cncr.21107. PMID: 15912493.

Linus Carl Pauling (1901–1994), recipient of two Nobel prizes, popularised the regular intake of vitamin C. He published two studies of vitamin C in end-stage cancer patients; their results apparently showed that vitamin C quadrupled survival times. A re-evaluation of these data, however, found that the vitamin C groups were less sick on entry to the study. Later clinical trials concluded that there was no benefit to high-dose vitamin C.

A 2010 survey of SCAM practitioners showed that they regularly use vitamin C injections for treating infection, cancer, and fatigue. Of 9328 patients for whom data was available, 101 had adverse effects, mostly minor, including lethargy/fatigue, change in mental status and vein irritation/phlebitis in 6 patients; but two deaths had also been reported. The authors of this paper conclude that *high dose IV vitamin C is in unexpectedly wide use by CAM practitioners. Other than the known complications of IV vitamin C in those with renal impairment or glucose 6 phosphate dehydrogenase deficiency, high dose intravenous vitamin C appears to be remarkably safe. Physicians should inquire about IV vitamin C use in patients with cancer, chronic, untreatable, or intractable conditions and be observant of unexpected harm, drug interactions, or benefit.*[91]

Vitamin C is a water-soluble antioxidant and acts as a cofactor for a large number of enzymes. While basic research in this area is buoyant and suggests that vitamin C might have some anti-cancer activity, controlled clinical trials testing its effectiveness as a cancer cure remain scarce.

- One hundred and fifty patients with advanced cancer participated in a controlled double-blind study to evaluate the effects of high-dose vitamin C on symptoms and survival. Patients were divided randomly into a group that received vitamin C (10 g per day) and one that received a comparably flavoured lactose placebo. Sixty evaluable patients received vitamin C and 63 received a placebo. Both groups were similar in age, sex, site of primary tumour, performance score, tumour grade and previous chemotherapy. The two groups showed no appreciable difference in changes in symptoms, performance status, appetite or weight. The median survival for all patients was about seven weeks, and the survival curves essentially overlapped. In this selected group of patients, we were unable to show a therapeutic benefit of high-dose vitamin C treatment.[92]

[91] Padayatty SJ, Sun AY, Chen Q, Espey MG, Drisko J, Levine M. Vitamin C: intravenous use by complementary and alternative medicine practitioners and adverse effects. PLoS One. 2010 July 7;5(7):e11414. http://doi.org/10.1371/journal.pone.0011414. PMID: 20628650; PMCID: PMC2898816.

[92] Creagan ET, Moertel CG, O'Fallon JR, Schutt AJ, O'Connell MJ, Rubin J, Frytak S. Failure of high-dose vitamin C (ascorbic acid) therapy to benefit patients with advanced cancer. A controlled

- In a double-blind study, 100 patients with advanced colorectal cancer were randomly assigned to treatment with either high-dose vitamin C (10 g daily) or placebo. Overall, these patients were in very good general condition, with minimal symptoms. None had received any previous treatment with cytotoxic drugs. Vitamin C therapy showed no advantage over placebo therapy with regard to either the interval between the beginning of treatment and disease progression or patient survival. Among patients with measurable disease, none had objective improvement. On the basis of this and our previous randomized study, it can be concluded that high-dose vitamin C therapy is not effective against advanced malignant disease regardless of whether the patient has had any prior chemotherapy.[93]
- An RCT included 27 patients with newly diagnosed stage III/IV ovarian cancer who received either conventional paclitaxel/carboplatin therapy alone (control group), or combined with intravenous vitamin C (treatment group). Addition of intravenous high-dose vitamin C was found to reduce toxicities associated with chemotherapy but the study was too small for assessing cancer survival times.[94]
- Another RCT with 20 patients undergoing multimodal treatment for oesophageal adenocarcinoma compared vitamin C (1000 mg/day) orally for 4 weeks with no supplementation. The results showed that vitamin C supplementation had a mildly protective effect in modulating regulators of inflammation and carcinogenesis. The trial did not report survival data.[95]

A 2015 systematic review failed to arrive at a positive conclusion.[96] Here is its abstract in full:

trial. N Engl J Med. 1979 Sept 27;301(13):687–90. http://doi.org/10.1056/NEJM19790927301 1303. PMID: 384241.

[93] Moertel CG, Fleming TR, Creagan ET, Rubin J, O'Connell MJ, Ames MM. High-dose vitamin C versus placebo in the treatment of patients with advanced cancer who have had no prior chemotherapy. A randomized double-blind comparison. N Engl J Med. 1985 Jan 17;312(3):137–41. http://doi.org/10.1056/NEJM198501173120301. PMID: 3880867.

[94] Ma Y, Chapman J, Levine M, Polireddy K, Drisko J, Chen Q. High-dose parenteral ascorbate enhanced chemosensitivity of ovarian cancer and reduced toxicity of chemotherapy. Sci Transl Med. 2014 Feb 5;6(222):222ra18. http://doi.org/10.1126/scitranslmed.3007154. PMID: 24500406.

[95] Abdel-Latif MMM, Babar M, Kelleher D, Reynolds JV. A pilot study of the impact of Vitamin C supplementation with neoadjuvant chemoradiation on regulators of inflammation and carcinogenesis in esophageal cancer patients. J Cancer Res Ther. 2019 Jan–Mar;15(1):185–191. http://doi.org/10.4103/jcrt.JCRT_763_16. PMID: 30880777.

[96] Jacobs C, Hutton B, Ng T, Shorr R, Clemons M. Is there a role for oral or intravenous ascorbate (vitamin C) in treating patients with cancer? A systematic review. Oncologist. 2015 Feb;20(2):210–23. http://doi.org/10.1634/theoncologist.2014-0381. Epub 2015 Jan 19. PMID: 25601965; PMCID: PMC4319640.

Background: Many cancer patients receive supplemental ascorbate (vitamin C) in the belief that it synergizes the anticancer effects of chemotherapy and reduces its toxicity.

Methods: A systematic review was performed to evaluate the antitumor effects and toxicity of ascorbate treatment. Medline (1946 to March 2014), EMBASE (1947 to March 2014), and the Cochrane central register (1993 to March 2014) were searched for randomized and observational studies.

Results: Of 696 identified records, 61 full-text articles were screened and 34 were included. In total, 5 randomized controlled trials (RCTs) ($n = 322$), 12 phase I/II trials ($n = 287$), 6 observational studies ($n = 7599$), and 11 case reports ($n = 267$) were identified. Because of study heterogeneity, no meta-analyses were performed. No RCTs reported any statistically significant improvements in overall or progression-free survival or reduced toxicity with ascorbate relative to control arm. Evidence for ascorbate's antitumor effects was limited to case reports and observational and uncontrolled studies.

Conclusion: There is no high-quality evidence to suggest that ascorbate supplementation in cancer patients either enhances the antitumor effects of chemotherapy or reduces its toxicity. Given the high financial and time costs to patients of this treatment, high-quality placebo-controlled trials are needed.

These findings were also confirmed in a 2019 review which did *not prove that there is a clinically relevant positive effect of vitamin C supplementation in cancer patients in general on the overall survival, clinical status, quality of life (QOL) and performance status (PS), since the quality of the studies published is low.*[97]

It follows that, despite the many rumour to the contrary, there is no good evidence to show that vitamin C is an effective cancer cure.

Plausibility	👎
Effectiveness	👎
Safety	👍
Cost	👍
Risk/benefit balance	👎

---

[97] van Gorkom GNY, Lookermans EL, Van Elssen CHMJ, Bos GMJ. The Effect of Vitamin C (Ascorbic Acid) in the Treatment of Patients with Cancer: A Systematic Review. Nutrients. 2019 Apr 28;11(5):977. http://doi.org/10.3390/nu11050977. PMID: 31035414; PMCID: PMC6566697.

Vitamin D

Vitamin D comprises a group of fat-soluble vitamins that is responsible for increasing intestinal absorption of calcium, magnesium, and phosphate. The most important vitamins D are vitamin D3 (cholecalciferol) and vitamin D2 (ergocalciferol). Being fat-soluble means it can accumulate in the body when over-dosed and cause symptoms known as hypervitaminosis D.

Clinical evidence that vitamin D might improve survival of cancer patients has been accumulating. A meta-analyses of observational studies suggested that higher blood 25-hydroxyvitamin D levels in cancer patients were associated with lower cancer-specific and overall mortalities. More importantly, a meta-analyses of RCTs confirmed that vitamin D supplementation improved survival. However, each single RCT failed to show statistical significance in the primary results.

In other words, while there are some encouraging data, compelling evidence that vitamin D supplementation effectively improves survival of patients with cancer is lacking.[98]

Plausibility	👍
Effectiveness	👎
Safety	👎
Cost	👍
Risk/benefit balance	👎

Comment

The evidence discussed above fails to show that any non-herbal supplement can be characterised as an effective cancer cure. Melatonin and vitamin D both might seem promising, and research in these areas should of course

[98] Akutsu T, Kitamura H, Himeiwa S, Kitada S, Akasu T, Urashima M. Vitamin D and Cancer Survival: Does Vitamin D Supplementation Improve the Survival of Patients with Cancer? Curr Oncol Rep. 2020 June 4;22(6):62. http://doi.org/10.1007/s11912-020-00929-4. PMID: 32495112.

continue. If it eventually does generate convincing evidence, these supplements would automatically cease to be a SCAM and become part of conventional oncology. This would be yet further confirmation of the point I have made repeatedly: an alternative cancer cure is a contradiction in terms.

3.5   Other Treatments

There are numerous SCAM cancer cures that cannot easily be put in any of the above categories but are sufficiently popular to deserve a mention in this book. This chapter is aimed at briefly discussing some of them.

Burzynski Regimen

Stanislaw Burzynski, M.D., a Polish-trained physician who immigrated to the US, isolated peptides from the urine of healthy individuals which he called antineoplastons. He claimed that these compounds would provide a protection against cancer and produced synthetic versions of them. In 1977, he opened a clinic in Houston, Texas, where he has ever since has been treating cancer patients with his oral antineoplaston therapy.

Burzynski believes antineoplastons are part of our natural defence system that helps prevent abnormal cell growth. He suggests that the reason some people develop cancer is a shortage of antineoplastons. By supplementing antineoplastons, Burzynski claims to turn cancer cells into healthy cells or to cause cancer cells to die without affecting healthy cells.

Bruzynski and his team have published around 50 articles on antineoplastons. These papers relate mostly to pre-clinical research, case reports or observational studies without control groups. Here is one typical example from 1977:

> Twenty-one patients with advanced cancer or leukemia were treated with antineoplaston A and followed for up to nine months. Dosage by intravenous, intramuscular, subcutaneous, rectal, intrapleural, intravesical and/or topical administration ranged from 0.6 to 33 $U/m^2/24$ h. Treatment was well tolerated, although side effects included fever of short duration and elevation of platelet and white blood count. In 18 cases some degree of clinical improvement was observed. Complete remission occurred in 4 cases. More than 50% remission occurred in 4 other cases which, along with another 6 cases, are continuing the treatment with high doses of antineoplaston A and show a continuing regression of the tumours although not yet achieving the criteria for complete remission; 2 of these 6 cases seem unlikely to achieve remission.

Two patients temporarily discontinued treatment. During treatment, 5 patients expired; in 2 of them, however, was seen significant regression of the neoplastic process. The deaths were not due to cancer or to any toxicity incurred by the treatment.[99]

More than 40 years later, no rigorously controlled clinical trials have emerged to support the assumption that antineoplastons are effective for curing any type of cancer. Thus it is fair to say that there is no good evidence to show that antineoplastons are an effective cure of any type of cancer.

Plausibility	👎
Effectiveness	👎
Safety	👎
Cost	👎
Risk/benefit balance	👎

Di Bella

The Di Bella multitherapy is a multidrug, custom made SCAM developed by Luigi Di Bella, an Italian physician, who claims his approach is effective in curing most cancers. The therapy consists of a (slightly variable) combination of the following drugs:

- melatonin (20 mg),
- bromocriptine (2.5 mg),
- somatostatin (3 mg) or octreotide (1 mg),
- retinoids (7 g),
- hydroxyurea (1 mg/day), only for glioblastoma,
- cyclophosphamide (50 mg/day),
- ascorbic acid (1–2 g),
- dihydrotachisterol (0.4–0.9 mg).

---

[99] Burzynski SR, Stolzmann Z, Szopa B, Stolzmann E, Kaltenberg OP. Antineoplaston A in cancer therapy. (I). Physiol Chem Phys. 1977;9(6):485–500. PMID: 275868.

In the late 1990s, the Di Bella therapy gained such popularity that the Italian authorities came under pressure to sponsor studies of it. Thus 11 studies were initiated. Their findings were published in one single paper; here is its abstract[100]:

Objective: To determine whether the treatment known as Di Bella multi-therapy exerts antitumour activity worthy of further controlled clinical evaluation.

Design: 11 independent multicentre uncontrolled phase II trials relevant to 8 different types of cancer.

Setting: 26 Italian hospitals specialising in cancer treatment.

Subjects: 386 patients with advanced cancer were enrolled in the trials between March and July 1998 and followed to 31 October 1998.

Interventions: Melatonin, bromocriptine, either somatostatin or octreotide, and retinoid solution, the drugs that constitute Di Bella multitherapy, were given to patients daily. Cyclophosphamide and hydroxyurea were added in some trials.

Main outcome measures: Responses were assessed every 1, 2, or 3 months, depending on the specific trial, and toxicity was evaluated using criteria developed by the World Health Organisation.

Results: No patient showed complete remission. Three patients showed partial remission: 1 of the 32 patients with non-Hodgkin's lymphoma; 1 of the 33 patients with breast cancer; and 1 of the 29 patients with pancreatic cancer. At the second examination, 12% (47) of the patients had stable disease; 52% (199) progressed; and 25% (97) died.

Conclusions: Di Bella multitherapy did not show sufficient efficacy in patients with advanced cancer to warrant further clinical testing.

Even though Di Bella published several further investigations,[101] there is still no sound evidence that this treatment is effective in curing any type of cancer.

Plausibility	
Effectiveness	

(continued)

---

[100] Italian Study Group for the Di Bella Multitherapy Trials. Evaluation of an unconventional cancer treatment (the Di Bella multitherapy): results of phase II trials in Italy. Italian Study Group for the Di Bella Multitherapy Trails. BMJ. 1999 Jan 23;318(7178):224–8. PMID: 9915729; PMCID: PMC27702.

[101] Di Bella G, Colori B, Mascia F. The Di Bella Method (DBM) improved survival, objective response and performance status in a retrospective observational clinical study on 55 cases of lymphomas. Neuro Endocrinol Lett. 2012;33(8):773–81. PMID: 23391973.

(continued)

Safety	👎
Cost	👎
Risk/benefit balance	👎

Factor AF2

Factor AF2 was developed in the 1940s and is a mixture of liver and spleen cells from sheep embryos. It is claimed to act as an immune stimulant and thus supposed to improve the prognosis of most cancers. The treatment has been tested in several clinical trials. Their findings fail to show that Factor AF2 changes the natural history of cancers. Here is the abstract of the most rigorous of these studies[102]:

This is a prospective randomized multicenter trial for evaluation of the biological response modifier Factor AF2 in advanced urothelial cancer treated with chemotherapy. Main aim of the study was the analysis of supportive effects. Additionally, patients were examined with regard to tumour response, time to progression and survival. 106 patients with advanced urothelial cancer received chemotherapy with cisplatin and methotrexate. They were randomized for additional Factor AF2 (500 mg i.v., given at days 0–3, 7–10 and 11–14). Myelotoxicity was more common and severe in the group without Factor AF2 reaching statistical significance. Gastrointestinal side effects occurred in both groups, though grade III to IV toxicity was more common without Factor AF2. Overall remission rate was 38%, median survival 33 weeks, mean time to progression 20 weeks. There was no significant difference between the two groups with or without Factor AF2.

This means that, despite the many claims to the contrary, there is no sound evidence to show that AF2 is an effective cancer cure.

---

[102] Krege S, Hinke A, Otto T, Rübben H. Bewertung des Komplementärtherapeutikums Factor AF2 als Supportivum in der Behandlung des fortgeschrittenen Urothelkarzinoms. Prospektiv randomisierte Multicenterstudie [Evaluation of the complementary drug Factor AF2 as a supportive agent in management of advanced urothelial carcinoma. Prospective randomized multicenter study]. Urologe A. 2002 Mar;41(2):164–8. German. http://doi.org/10.1007/s001200100129. PMID: 11993095.

Plausibility	👎
Effectiveness	👎
Safety	👎
Cost	👎
Risk/benefit balance	👎

Gonzalez Regimen

The Gonzalez regimen is a treatment based on the obsolete ideas of James Beard, a Scottish physician, who believed that pancreatic enzymes control cancer cells. It is claimed to work in three different ways:

1. It is supposed to detoxify the body.
2. It allegedly supports the autonomous nervous system.
3. It is said to stimulate the immune defence.

The regimen includes consuming enzymes (Sect. 3.4), a staggering amount of diverse dietary supplements such as vitamins and minerals (patients following the regimen need to swallow ~200 pills daily), coffee enemas and a individualized diet consisting mainly of organic foods.

Dr Nicolas Gonzalez studied his regimen in 11 patients who had advanced pancreatic cancer. In 1993, he reported selected results of the study to the National Cancer Institute (NCI). They suggested that patients treated with the Gonzalez regimen lived a median of 17 months, which is longer than usual for patients with this disease. A subsequent 7-year controlled clinical trial included patients who had stage 2–4 pancreatic cancer. In this study, one group of patients followed the Gonzalez regimen while the control group was given standard treatment of chemotherapy. The results showed that *among patients who have pancreatic cancer, those who chose gemcitabine-based chemotherapy survived more than three times as long (14.0 v 4.3 months) and had better quality of life than those who chose proteolytic enzyme treatment.*[103]

---

[103] Chabot JA, Tsai WY, Fine RL, Chen C, Kumah CK, Antman KA, Grann VR. Pancreatic proteolytic enzyme therapy compared with gemcitabine-based chemotherapy for the treatment of pancreatic

The few studies of the Gonzalez regimen have recently been reviewed, and the conclusion was not encouraging: *No data concerning the effectiveness of the Gonzalez regimen for the treatment of cancer patients with other types of cancer have been reported, despite claims that a variety of cancers can be treated. In addition, there is no safety or efficacy information on the regimen in children. No clinical trials of this regimen have been conducted in children, and this extremely difficult regimen may be prohibitive in young children.*[104]

It is therefore indisputable that the Gonzalez regimen lacks good evidence of effectiveness as a cancer cure.

Plausibility	👎
Effectiveness	👎
Safety	👎
Cost	👎
Risk/benefit balance	👎

Hulda Clark

Hulda Clark (1928–2009) was a Canadian naturopath who believed that cancer (and several other diseases) was caused by an intestinal parasite. To eliminate the infestation, patients needed to buy her 'zapper', a device that used a weak electrical current and allegedly killed the bug.

These assumptions are amongst the least plausible in all of SCAM. Perhaps for this reason, there is not a single clinical trial testing the effectiveness of this approach.

Plausibility	👎
Effectiveness	👎

(continued)

cancer. J Clin Oncol. 2010 Apr 20;28(12):2058–63. http://doi.org/10.1200/JCO.2009.22.8429. Epub 2009 Aug 17. PMID: 19687327; PMCID: PMC2860407.

[104] PDQ Integrative, Alternative, and Complementary Therapies Editorial Board. Gonzalez Regimen (PDQ®): Health Professional Version. 2018 Aug 22. In: PDQ Cancer Information Summaries [Internet]. Bethesda (MD): National Cancer Institute (US); 2002. Available from: https://www.ncbi.nlm.nih.gov/books/NBK65848/.

(continued)

Safety	👎
Cost	👎
Risk/benefit balance	👎

Hydrazine Sulphate

In the 1970s, Dr. Joseph Gold postulated that hydrazine sulphate was a powerful anti-cancer drug. He claimed that hydrazine sulphate limits the ability of cancer cells to obtain glucose and thus energy for survival. Gold later published case series to support his assumption[105]:

> In a series of 84 various evaluable disseminated cancer patients treated with hydrazine sulfate as a result of a pharmaceutical-sponsored investigational new drug (IND) study, it was found that 59/84 or 70% of the cases improved subjectively and 14/84 or 17% improved objectively. Subjective responses included increased appetite with either weight gain or cessation of weight loss, increase in strength and improved performance status and decrease in pain. Objective responses included measurable tumour regression, disappearance of or decrease in neoplastic-associated disorders and long-term (over 1 year) 'stabilized condition'. Of the overall 59 subjective improvements 25 (42%) had no concurrent or prior (within 3 months) anticancer therapy of any type. Of the 14 objective improvements 7 (50%) had no concurrent or prior anticancer therapy. Of the remaining cases in which there was either concurrent or prior anticancer therapy, improvements occurred only after the addition of hydrazine sulfate to the treatment regimen. Duration of improvement was variable, from temporary to long-term and continuing. Side effects were mild, comprising for the most part low incidences of extremity paresthesias, nausea, pruritus and drowsiness; there was no indication of bone marrow depression.

---

[105] Gold J. Use of hydrazine sulfate in terminal and preterminal cancer patients: results of investigational new drug (IND) study in 84 evaluable patients. Oncology. 1975;32(1):1–10. http://doi.org/10.1159/000225043. PMID: 1208024.

These findings motivated several other researchers to test Gold's hypothesis. None of the subsequent studies confirmed Gold's findings.[106] [107] A review of the totality of the evidence concluded that *the value of hydrazine sulfate as an antitumour agent—specifically its capacity to stabilize tumour size, cause tumour regression and improve survival—remains uncertain.*[108]

Hydrazine sulphate is therefore not a SCAM that cures cancer of any type.

Plausibility	👎
Effectiveness	👎
Safety	🤚
Cost	👍
Risk/benefit balance	👎

Kelley Protocol

Dr. William Donald Kelley (1925–2005), a US dentist, was diagnosed with metastatic pancreatic cancer and survived using the Gerson approach (Sect. 3.3) in combination with pancreatic enzyme therapy, often called "non-specific metabolic therapy". The Kelly protocol is based on the belief that wrong foods cause cancer to grow, while the right foods allow natural body defences to work. In 1969, Kelly published his story and an assumed explanation of why his protocol worked, entitled *One Answer to Cancer*.[109]

Kelley claimed a 93% success rate for cancer patients who came to him before trying conventional treatments, and a 50% chance of survival even for end-stage cancer patients. In 1976, the Texas Dental Board suspended

[106] Kosty MP, Fleishman SB, Herndon JE 2nd, Coughlin K, Kornblith AB, Scalzo A, Morris JC, Mortimer J, Green MR. Cisplatin, vinblastine, and hydrazine sulfate in advanced, non-small-cell lung cancer: a randomized placebo-controlled, double-blind phase III study of the Cancer and Leukemia Group B. J Clin Oncol. 1994 June;12(6):1113–20. http://doi.org/10.1200/JCO.1994.12.6.1113. PMID: 8201372.

[107] Loprinzi CL, Goldberg RM, Su JQ, Mailliard JA, Kuross SA, Maksymiuk AW, Kugler JW, Jett JR, Ghosh C, Pfeifle DM, et al. Placebo-controlled trial of hydrazine sulfate in patients with newly diagnosed non-small-cell lung cancer. J Clin Oncol. 1994 June;12(6):1126–9. http://doi.org/10.1200/JCO.1994.12.6.1126. PMID: 8201374.

[108] Kaegi E. Unconventional therapies for cancer: 4. Hydrazine sulfate. Task Force on Alternative Therapies of the Canadian Breast Cancer Research Initiative. CMAJ. 1998 May 19;158(10):1327–30. PMID: 9614826; PMCID: PMC1229327.

[109] http://www.drkelley.com/CANLIVER55.html#_Toc434239866.

his license for 5 years for providing "non-dental" cancer therapies. He then moved his practice to Tijuana, Mexico.

The actor Steve McQueen, in the advanced stages of mesothelioma, turned to Kelly in search of a cure. McQueen died despite Kelley's treatments. In turn, Kelley claimed that he had, in fact, successfully cured McQueen, but that the medical establishment subsequently had McQueen murdered in order to prevent him "blowing the lid off the cancer racket."

To date, there is no sound evidence that the Kelly protocol is an effective cure for any type of cancer.

Plausibility	👎
Effectiveness	👎
Safety	👎
Cost	👎
Risk/benefit balance	👎

Naturopathy

Naturopathy is an eclectic system of healthcare that employs elements of both SCAM and conventional medicine to support the body's own self-healing capacity. Naturopaths predominantly use treatments based on therapeutic options that are thought of as natural, e. g. naturally occurring substances such as herbs, as well as water, exercise, diet, fresh air, pressure, heat and cold—but occasionally also acupuncture, homeopathy and manual therapies.

In many countries, naturopathy is not a protected title; this means your naturopaths may have some training, but this might not be obligatory. Medical doctors can, of course, also practice naturopathy. Some countries allow the titles 'doctors of naturopathy' or 'naturopathic physicians'; these practitioners tend to see themselves as primary care physicians even though they have not been to medical school.[110] [111]

[110] Smith MJ, Logan AC. Naturopathy. Med Clin North Am. 2002 Jan;86(1):173–84. http://doi.org/10.1016/s0025-7125(03)00079-8. PMID: 11795088.
[111] Atwood KC 4th. Naturopathy: a critical appraisal. MedGenMed. 2003 Dec 30;5(4):39. PMID: 14745386.

Naturopathy is steeped in the obsolete concept of vitalism, i.e. the belief that living organisms are fundamentally different from non-living entities because they contain some non-physical element or are governed by different principles than are inanimate things. Naturopathic treatment modalities include:

- diet and clinical nutrition,
- behavioural change,
- hydrotherapy,
- homeopathy,
- botanical medicine,
- physical medicine,
- pharmaceuticals,
- minor surgery (see Footnote 110).

Naturopathy is implicitly based on the assumption that natural means safe. This notion is demonstrably wrong and misleading: not all the treatments used by naturopaths are natural, and hardly any are totally free of risks. Naturopaths tend to believe they can cure most diseases, including cancer. The 2019 'Oncology Association of Naturopathic Physicians: Principles of Care Guidelines' state that b*ecause of their training as primary care providers delivering whole-person care …* *can play an important role in the care of cancer patients.*[112] A 2019 survey from Canada revealed the 10 most frequently considered natural health products used by naturopaths to treat childhood cancer:

- fish-derived omega-3 fatty acid (83%),
- vitamin D (83%),
- probiotics (82%),
- melatonin (74%),
- vitamin C (73%),
- homeopathic Arnica (69%),
- turmeric/curcumin (68%),
- glutamine (67%),
- Astragalus membranaceus (64%),
- Coriolus versicolor/PSK (polysaccharide K) extracts (62%).

And the top five nutritional recommendations were:

- anti-inflammatory diets (78%),

---

[112] Curr Oncol. 2019 Feb; 26(1): 12–18. Published online 2019 Feb 1. http://doi.org/10.3747/co.26.4815.

- dairy restriction (66%),
- Mediterranean diet (66%),
- gluten restriction (62%),
- and ketogenic diet (57%).

The authors concluded that *the results of our clinical practice survey highlight naturopathic interventions across four domains with a strong rationale for further inquiry in the care of children with cancer.*[113]

From the previous chapters, it seems clear that none of the naturopathic treatments have been proven to be effective cures for any type of cancer. It follows that there is little sound evidence that naturopathy might offer an effective option to cure cancer.

Plausibility	👎
Effectiveness	👎
Safety	👎
Cost	👎
Risk/benefit balance	👎

German New Medicine

German New Medicine (GNM) is the creation of Ryke Geerd Hamer (1935–2017), a German doctor. The name is oddly reminiscent of the 'Neue Deutsche Heilkunde' created by the Nazis during the Third Reich. According to GNM's proponents, every disease, in particular cancer, is triggered by an isolating and shocking event, GNM assists in identifying that shocking moment in our lives that preceded the cancer and in turn allowing our bodies to complete its natural healing cycle back to full health.[114] Hamer believed to have discovered the '5 laws of nature':

1. The Iron Rule of Cancer
2. The two-phased development of disease

[113] Psihogios A, Ennis JK, Seely D. Naturopathic Oncology Care for Pediatric Cancers: A Practice Survey. Integr Cancer Ther. 2019 Jan–Dec;18:1534735419878504. http://doi.org/10.1177/153473 5419878504. PMID: 31566009; PMCID: PMC6769230.

[114] http://www.gnmtherapy.co.uk/about-the-gnm/.

3. Ontogenetic system of tumours and cancer equivalent diseases
4. Ontogenetic system of microbes
5. Nature's biological meaning of a disease.

Hamer also postulated that:

- All diseases are caused by psychological conflicts.
- Conventional medicine is a conspiracy of Jews to decimate the non-Jewish population.
- Microbes do not cause diseases.
- AIDS is just an allergy.
- Cancer is the result of a mental shock.

None of Hamer's assumptions are plausible or based on facts. There is no sound evidence that GNM is effective for any type of cancer. Several deaths have been associated with Hamer's approach. [e. g.115]

Plausibility	👎
Effectiveness	👎
Safety	👎
Cost	👎
Risk/benefit balance	👎

Powerlight

Powerlight is a relatively new SCAM that is being promoted against many serious diseases, including cancer. Here is what the website[116] states about it:

> The very word "cancer" for patients is such a heavy burden, that psychological support actually is necessary when a patient gets such a diagnosis. In this section, we are pleased and proud to set an end to this terrifying illness.

---

[115] https://derstandard.at/2000043742380/18-Jaehrige-starbEltern-verweigerten-krebskranker-Tochter-Therapie.
[116] http://www.powerlight-dubai.com/powerlight-ca.html.

A lot of different tumours in current language are called cancer. A cancer is based on epithelian tissue. This tissue occurs in different organs. Because of that we find this tumour: as an

- Anal carcinoma
- Bronchial carcinoma
- Testicle carcinoma
- Laryngeal cancer
- Colon cancer
- Oesophageal cancer
- Gastric cancer
- Breast cancer
- Kidney carcinoma
- Ovary carcinoma
- Pancreas carcinoma
- Pharynx (throat) carcinoma
- Prostate carcinoma

Cancer is one of the most dreaded diseases we know.

We found the possibility to heal every kind of cancer, anyway what staging the tumour has. Also, patients in the final stadium feel better after the third ampoule* and will be healed completely. The first ampoule brings a patient a better psychic situation.

For other tumours we have special medicines in our product list. Before taking Powerlight medicine it is necessary to have an exact diagnosis from a hospital. For example, it was necessary to develop against carcinomas in the childhood other cluster structures—this is now our drug KIC. Tumours spreading from other tissues are to be treated with Powerlight NR, Powerlight H+NH and Powerlight LE.

If a patient started his treatment with conventional chemotherapy, the side effects will be bettered, when the patient gets Powerlight EG. The intake of Powerlight CA and Powerlight EG in the same period is not possible. In serious cases, it has to be proved, whether the dangerous situation is caused primarily by the tumour or by the chemotherapy. According to this, the heaviest burden has to be treated first.

All tumours that are not cancers, will not be healed by Powerlight CA. In these cases find an other correct medicine under "Product list" in this homepage.

The website also provides the answer to the question how powerlight works:

The scientific background of our products is the physics of antimatter. With the help of positron radiation we can represent order patterns of living matter. Antimatter is able to copy patterns of organisms, when we put them into the electromagnetic field of antimatter. Such patterns show irregularities in the living matter. Normally living matter is structured by strict order patterns. The irregularities are causes of illness. Powerlight reconditions order patterns of living systems because these order patterns also by heavy illnesses are not destroyed but only overlapped. The original order patterns are guide rails of the electron transfer by Clusters.

It has been reported that POWERLIGHT and some of the practitioners offering it are being sued in Austria after several cancer patients died.[117] There is no evidence that this therapy has any effects on cancer or other diseases.

Plausibility	👎
Effectiveness	👎
Safety	👍
Cost	👎
Risk/benefit balance	👎

Comment

The notion of an effective SCAM cancer therapy is a contradiction in terms. Either a treatment is an effective cancer cure, or it is not. If it works, it belongs to conventional oncology, if not it should be discarded. If a SCAM does show promise, it would be researched rigorously and tested scientifically; during this process it would become a conventional treatment. Shark cartilage is an apt example (Sect. 3.4). On the basis of the (incorrect) notion that sharks do not get cancer, it was is heavily promoted as a SCAM cancer cure. In-vitro tests even demonstrated that shark cartilage has anti-angiogenic activity. Such findings made the sales figures rocket and subsequently the two shark species used for the commercial preparations were driven to the brink of extinction. Finally, a clinical trial of shark cartilage demonstrated that our hopes were in vain. The story confirms that regular scientists and conventional oncologists are keen to find new anticancer drugs and they do not care from what source they originate. This argument is further strengthened by the fact that it has

---

[117] https://medwatch.de/2020/05/15/warten-auf-ein-wunder/.

happened before: numerous modern cancer drugs, e.g. Taxol, were originally derived from plants.

All this should just be common sense. Yet, a strange sort of paranoia stubbornly persists in the realm of SCAM. Many believe that mainstream oncology and 'big pharma' conspire to actively suppress the fact that shark cartilage, Laetrile, the Gerson diet, Essiac, etc., could save thousands of lives of cancer patients. Sometimes this is even supported by statements from VIPs; Prince Charles, for instance, told us some time ago in no uncertain terms about the virtues of the Gerson diet as a cure for cancer (see foreword by M. Baum).[118]

In the final analysis, the myth of a SCAM cancer cure assumes that scientists are sadistic misfits without morals, ethics or a conscience who would forfeit a promising option simply because it did not originate from their ranks. Such notions are naïve and insulting to those who dedicate their lives to making progress in cancer care and do not improve the cooperation between oncologists and SCAM practitioners.

The evidence laid out in this chapter clearly shows that the assumption of a SCAM cancer cure is unrealistic and counter-productive. As we will see in the following chapter, this does, however, not mean that SCAM has no role at all to play in helping cancer patients.

---

[118] Baum M. An open letter to the Prince of Wales: with respect, your highness, you've got it wrong. BMJ 2004; 329:118.

4

Palliative and Supportive Care

In the previous chapter, we have seen that virtually no SCAM promoted as cancer cures is supported by sound evidence. This lack of proven effectiveness renders them dangerous to any cancer patient who decides to try them. If cancer patients use a SCAM to cure cancer while forfeiting conventional treatments, this choice would almost certainly cause significant harm and, in dramatic cases, it can even hasten their death. But this warning does not mean that SCAM has nothing to offer for cancer patients. As we will see in this chapter, some forms of SCAM show considerable promise in supportive and palliative care of cancer patients.

The treatments employed in supportive and palliative care have fundamentally different aims from the therapies used as cancer cures: they do not claim to change the natural history of the disease, their goal is to improve cancer patients' quality of life by alleviating the suffering of cancer patients. A supportive or palliative therapy is thus defined by the way it is used and not by the nature of the treatment; one specific SCAM might be advocated as a cure (without good evidence, as we have seen in the previous chapter) and also used in supportive and palliative care. This means that some SCAMs which we have already encountered in the previous chapter will be re-discussed from a different perspective in this chapter.

Supportive and palliative care is usually teamwork that might involve oncologists, general practitioners, cares, SCAM practitioners, the patient's family and others. It is focussed not just on physical symptoms but also

E. Ernst, *So-Called Alternative Medicine (SCAM) for Cancer*, https://doi.org/10.1007/978-3-030-74158-7_4

on psychosocial problems. It can be aimed at the following complaints commonly encountered in cancer care:

- Anxiety
- Appetite loss
- Constipation
- Depression
- Diarrhoea
- Dyspnoea
- Fatigue
- Incontinence
- Insomnia
- Irritability
- Nausea and vomiting
- Pain
- Skin irritation
- Swollen limb
- Weakness
- Weight loss.

These symptoms can be due to the disease, the treatments or they can relate to independent issues. Nausea can, for instance, be caused by chemotherapy, by surgery, or by a raised intracranial pressure due to a brain tumour. Dyspnoea can be due to fluid overload, pleural effusion, airway obstruction or cachexia. Perhaps the most common symptom to adversely affect the quality of life of cancer patients is pain. Pain specialists often differentiate between:

- Somatic pain which often occurs with bone metastases caused by the destruction and new formation of bone.
- Visceral pain originates from inner organs and can sometimes be experienced as referred pain at sites distant from the respective organ.
- Neuropathic pain results from injury to neural structures, often caused by chemotherapy.

The pain of cancer patients can have many different guises, including:

- Pain syndromes associated with tumour infiltration such as headache, cranial neuralgias, glossopharyngeal neuralgia, trigeminal neuralgia.
- Pain syndromes associated with cancer chemotherapy such as peripheral neuropathy, perineal pain, headache, mononeuropathy.

- Pain associated with surgery such as postmastectomy pain, pain after neck dissection, pain after thoracotomy, phantom limb pain.
- Pain associated with radiotherapy such as fibrosis of a nerve plexus or myelopathy.

The multidimensional nature of the many different cancer-related symptoms, their constantly changing patterns, the multifactorial aetiologic mechanisms and the multiple interactions between symptoms present major challenges to the team providing supportive and palliative cancer care. Both pharmacologic and non-pharmacologic approaches are required to best meet these challenges and find the optimal therapeutic approach.

In many cases, cancer is a chronic disease: cancer patients often live many years while experiencing a range of physical and psychological symptoms. To optimize the outcomes from supportive and palliative cancer care, numerous SCAMs are being recommended. However, these recommendations are often uncritical and not based on evidence. In this chapter, I will discuss the evidence for or against the most popular SCAMs used in supportive and palliative cancer care.

4.1 Acupuncture

Acupuncture is a therapy that typically involves sticking needles into special points on the skin. There is a multitude of acupuncture types; these points can allegedly be stimulated not just by inserting needles, but also with

- heat (moxibustion),
- electrical currents (electroacupuncture),
- ultrasound,
- pressure (acupressure),
- bee-stings (see apitherapy),
- injections (bio-puncture),
- light,
- colour, etc.

Then there is body acupuncture, ear acupuncture (auriculotherapy) and even tongue acupuncture. Some therapists employ the traditional Chinese approach, while so-called 'Western' acupuncturists adhere to the principles of conventional medicine. Traditional Chinese acupuncturists base their practice on the belief that acupuncture restores the balance between two life-forces, 'yin and yang'. In contrast, medical acupuncturists tend to cite neurophysiological theories as to how acupuncture might work[1]; even though these may appear plausible, they are mere theories and constitute no proof for acupuncture's validity. According to the traditional view, acupuncture is useful for virtually every condition and symptom affecting mankind. According to 'Western' acupuncturists, acupuncture is effective for a much smaller range of conditions, mostly chronic pain.

Acupuncture is being recommended for virtually any problem that cancer patients might experience. In the following section, I will discuss the evidence as it relates to acupuncture in the management of just those three specific symptoms of cancer patients for which there is ample evidence.

Pain

A 2012 systematic review included a total of 15 RCTs the majority of which suggested positive effects of acupuncture on cancer pain. However, most studies were flawed and the effects were small in comparison to those achievable with other therapeutic options. The conclusion was that *the total number of RCTs included in the analysis and their methodological quality was too low to draw firm conclusions.*[2] This verdict was further confirmed by a 2016 meta-analysis which showed that *acupuncture alone did not have superior pain-relieving effects as compared with conventional drug therapy.*[3]

A systematic review published in 2020 included 17 RCTs with a total of 1111 patients. Seven RCTs suggested that real acupuncture was associated with reduced pain intensity compared to sham acupuncture. The authors concluded that *acupuncture and/or acupressure was significantly associated with reduced cancer pain and decreased use of analgesics, although the evidence level was moderate. This finding suggests that more rigorous trials are needed to identify the association of acupuncture and acupressure with specific types of cancer pain*

[1] Zhao ZQ. Neural mechanism underlying acupuncture analgesia. Prog Neurobiol. 2008 Aug;85(4):355–75. https://doi.org/10.1016/j.pneurobio.2008.05.004. Epub 2008 Jun 5. PMID: 18582529.

[2] Choi TY, Lee MS, Kim TH, Zaslawski C, Ernst E. Acupuncture for the treatment of cancer pain: a systematic review of randomised clinical trials. Support Care Cancer. 2012 Jun;20(6):1147–58. https://doi.org/10.1007/s00520-012-1432-9. Epub 2012 Mar 25. PMID: 22447366.

[3] Hu C, Zhang H, Wu W, Yu W, Li Y, Bai J, Luo B, Li S. Acupuncture for Pain Management in Cancer: A Systematic Review and Meta-Analysis. Evid Based Complement Alternat Med. 2016;2016:1720239. https://doi.org/10.1155/2016/1720239. Epub 2016 Feb 10. PMID: 26977172; PMCID: PMC4764722.

and to integrate such evidence into clinical care to reduce opioid use.[4] Assessing this paper critically, it should, however, be noted that:

- About half of the primary studies are by Chinese investigators; such trials have repeatedly been noted to exclusively report positive results and be unreliable.[5]
- Many of these trials are published in Chinese and can thus not be checked by non-Chinese readers (nor, presumably, by many of the experts who acted as peer-reviewers).
- One paper included in the review is a mere doctoral thesis which usually is not peer-reviewed at all.
- The authors state that they included only clinical trials that compared acupuncture and acupressure with a sham control, analgesic therapy, or usual care. However, this is evidently not true; many of the studies followed an 'A+B versus B' design comparing acupuncture plus a conventional therapy against the conventional therapy. Such trials cannot produce a negative finding, even if 'A' is a placebo (Sect. 1.7).
- Contrary to what the authors claim, the quality of most of the included studies was extremely poor.
- One included paper is entitled 'Clinical observation on 30 cases of moderate and severe cancer pain of bone metastasis treated by auricular acupressure', yet the authors claim to have included only RCTs.

A more recent review confirmed that the evidence is weak and stressed that *low-level evidence adversely affects the reliability of findings.*[6]

Whichever way we turn the existing data, it seems clear that acupuncture is not as effective for alleviating cancer pain as acupuncturists try to make us believe and certainly not as effective as standard treatments for controlling cancer pain. Whether it might serve as an effective adjunct to conventional therapies is still a matter of debate.

---

[4] He Y, Guo X, May BH, Zhang AL, Liu Y, Lu C, Mao JJ, Xue CC, Zhang H. Clinical Evidence for Association of Acupuncture and Acupressure With Improved Cancer Pain: A Systematic Review and Meta-Analysis. JAMA Oncol. 2020 Feb 1;6(2):271–278. https://doi.org/10.1001/jamaoncol.2019. 5233. PMID: 31855257; PMCID: PMC6990758.

[5] Data fabrication in China is an 'open secret' (edzardernst.com).

[6] Yang J, Wahner-Roedler DL, Zhou X, Johnson LA, Do A, Pachman DR, Chon TY, Salinas M, Millstine D, Bauer BA. Acupuncture for palliative cancer pain management: systematic review. BMJ Support Palliat Care. 2021 Jan 13:bmjspcare-2020–002638. https://doi.org/10.1136/bmjspcare-2020-002638. Epub ahead of print. PMID: 33441387.

Nausea and Vomiting

Nausea and vomiting are common side effects of chemotherapy, radiotherapy or surgery. The problem can usually be successfully treated with standard anti-emetic drugs. Some patients, however, may not respond satisfactorily and others might prefer a drug-free option such as acupuncture or acupressure for which there has, indeed, been some encouraging evidence.

A large study assessed the effectiveness of self-administered acupressure using wristbands pressing the P6 point (anterior surface of the forearm), compared with sham acupressure wristbands and standard care alone in the management of chemotherapy-induced nausea. In total, 500 patients were included. The primary outcome analysis revealed that no significant differences were detected in relation to vomiting outcomes, anxiety and quality of life. The authors concluded that *no clear recommendations can be made about the use of acupressure wristbands in the management of chemotherapy-related nausea and vomiting.*[7]

The current Cochrane review concluded *that there is low-quality evidence supporting the use of PC6 acupoint stimulation over sham.*[8] And a systematic review specifically focussing on moxibustion concluded that *the evidence obtained is not sufficient because of the lack of strict clinical trials.*[9]

This means that the evidence is highly contradictory. If one critically analyses the primary studies, one finds that the more rigorous trials and those published by researchers who are free of conflicts of interest tend to produce negative findings. In essence, this suggests that the evidence is less than convincing.

Fatigue

Many cancer patients suffer from fatigue which sometimes can be severe or even debilitating. The exact causes of this common symptom are not

[7] Molassiotis A, Russell W, Hughes J, Breckons M, Lloyd-Williams M, Richardson J, Hulme C, Brearley SG, Campbell M, Garrow A, Ryder WD. The effectiveness of acupressure for the control and management of chemotherapy-related acute and delayed nausea: a randomized controlled trial. J Pain Symptom Manage. 2014 Jan;47(1):12–25. https://doi.org/10.1016/j.jpainsymman.2013.03.007. Epub 2013 Apr 17. PMID: 23602325.

[8] Lee A, Chan SKC, Fan LTY. Stimulation of the wrist acupuncture point PC6 for preventing postoperative nausea and vomiting. Cochrane Database of Systematic Reviews 2015, Issue 11. Art. No.: CD003281. https://doi.org/10.1002/14651858.CD003281.pub4.

[9] Huang Z, Qin Z, Yao Q, Wang Y, Liu Z. Moxibustion for Chemotherapy-Induced Nausea and Vomiting: A Systematic Review and Meta-Analysis. Evid Based Complement Alternat Med. 2017;2017:9854893. https://doi.org/10.1155/2017/9854893. Epub 2017 Oct 12. PMID: 29234451; PMCID: PMC5660813.

entirely clear. Most likely they relate to a combination of the cancer and the treatments used to cure it. Managing cancer-related fatigue (CRF) is thus an important part of the palliative and supportive care of cancer patients. Acupuncture is often advocated for this purpose and many centres currently use it routinely. But does it truly work?

A recent trial was aimed at assessing the effectiveness of maintenance acupuncture in the management of CRF; acupuncture or self-acupuncture/self-needling was compared with no such treatment. Breast cancer patients were randomized to receive:

- four weekly sessions of acupuncture delivered by an acupuncturist,
- four self-administered weekly acupuncture sessions (self-needling);
- or no acupuncture at all.

The primary outcome measure was general fatigue, while mood, quality of life and safety served as secondary endpoints. In total, 197 patients were randomized. The results failed to demonstrate significant inter-group differences in any of the parameters evaluated. The authors concluded that *maintenance acupuncture did not yield important improvements beyond those observed after an initial clinic-based course of acupuncture.*[10]

But this is just one of several available studies. If we want a fair verdict, we must of course consider the totality of the reliable evidence. The aim of our 2013 systematic review was to critically evaluate the effectiveness of acupuncture (AT) for CRF based on all the available studies. Seven RCTs met the eligibility criteria. Most were small pilot studies with serious methodological flaws. Four RCTs showed effectiveness of AT or AT in addition to usual care (UC) over sham AT, UC, enhanced UC, or no intervention for alleviating CRF. Three RCTs failed to demonstrate an effect of AT over sham treatment. It was concluded that *overall, the quantity and quality of RCTs included in the analysis were too low to draw meaningful conclusions. Even in the positive trials, it remained unclear whether the observed outcome was due to specific effects of AT or nonspecific effects of care.*[11]

However, a 2018 systematic review suggested that acupuncture has positive effects on fatigue in cancer patients, regardless of concurrent anti-cancer

[10] Molassiotis A, Bardy J, Finnegan-John J, Mackereth P, Ryder WD, Filshie J, Ream E, Eaton D, Richardson A. A randomized, controlled trial of acupuncture self-needling as maintenance therapy for cancer-related fatigue after therapist-delivered acupuncture. Ann Oncol. 2013 Jun;24(6):1645–52. https://doi.org/10.1093/annonc/mdt034. Epub 2013 Feb 21. PMID: 23436910.

[11] Posadzki P, Moon TW, Choi TY, Park TY, Lee MS, Ernst E. Acupuncture for cancer-related fatigue: a systematic review of randomized clinical trials. Support Care Cancer. 2013 Jul;21(7):2067–73. https://doi.org/10.1007/s00520-013-1765-z. Epub 2013 Feb 24. PMID: 23435597.

treatment, particularly among breast cancer patients. The meta-analysis also indicated that acupuncture could significantly mitigate CRF compared with sham acupuncture or usual care. The authors concluded that *acupuncture is effective for CRF management and should be recommended as a beneficial alternative therapy for CRF patients, particularly for breast cancer patients and those currently undergoing anti-cancer treatment.*[12]

The contradiction between the two reviews seems to be due to the methodological flaws in the primary studies. Depending on how critically they are evaluated, review authors arrive either at positive or negative conclusions about the effectiveness of acupuncture for fatigue. This essentially means that the value of acupuncture for supportive and palliative cancer care remains debatable.

Even though acupuncture is often considered to be free of serious adverse effects, it can cause life-threatening complications. Pneumothorax, infections, and cardiac tamponade have all been reported.[13]

As mentioned above, acupuncture has also been tested for a range of further cancer-related symptoms. In these cases, the evidence suffers from similar problems: there are only few studies, most are methodologically flawed, and their results are full of contradictions. Even outspoken proponents of acupuncture therefore admit *that the evidence for use of acupuncture to treat symptoms in palliative care patients is relatively weak.*[14] The overall conclusion thus is disappointing: evidence for acupuncture as an effective therapy in palliative and supportive cancer care is currently far from convincing.

Plausibility	👎
Effectiveness	👎 / 👍
Safety	👍 / 👍

(continued)

[12] Zhang Y, Lin L, Li H, Hu Y, Tian L. Effects of acupuncture on cancer-related fatigue: a meta-analysis. Support Care Cancer. 2018 Feb;26(2):415–425. https://doi.org/10.1007/s00520-017-3955-6. Epub 2017 Nov 11. PMID: 29128952.

[13] Ernst E, Lee MS, Choi TY. Acupuncture: does it alleviate pain and are there serious risks? A review of reviews. Pain. 2011 Apr;152(4):755–764. https://doi.org/10.1016/j.pain.2010.11.004. PMID: 21440191.

[14] Birch S, Bovey M, Alraek T, Robinson N, Kim TH, Lee MS. Acupuncture as a Treatment Within Integrative Health for Palliative Care: A Brief Narrative Review of Evidence and Recommendations. J Altern Complement Med. 2020 Sep;26(9):784–791. https://doi.org/10.1089/acm.2020.0032. PMID: 32924554.

(continued)

Cost	
Risk/benefit balance	

4.2   Massage

Massage is an ancient treatment that has long been part of most medical traditions. It typically involves the manual manipulation of the soft tissues below the skin. Various types and techniques of massage have emerged over the centuries. In this chapter, I will mention those massage and massage-related therapies that are often used in palliative and supportive cancer care.

Aromatherapy

Aromatherapy normally combines the application of diluted essential oils with a gentle massage. It seems reasonable to assume that most of the relaxing effects of aromatherapy are due to the gentle massage rather than any specific effects of the essential oils.

Aromatherapy is often considered to be devoid of risks. However, this assumption is not entirely correct. A review of the potential of harm concluded that *aromatherapy has the potential to cause adverse effects some of which are serious. Their frequency remains unknown.*[15]

It is claimed that cancer patients benefit from aromatherapy in various ways:

- reduced anxiety levels,
- relief of emotional stress,
- pain relief,
- reduction of fatigue.

The evidence, is, however, not clear-cut. Our own RCT of 2004, for instance, failed to yield positive effects of aromatherapy massage on the

---

[15] Posadzki P, Alotaibi A, Ernst E. Adverse effects of aromatherapy: a systematic review of case reports and case series. Int J Risk Saf Med. 2012 Jan 1;24(3):147–61. https://doi.org/10.3233/JRS-2012-0568. PMID: 22936057.

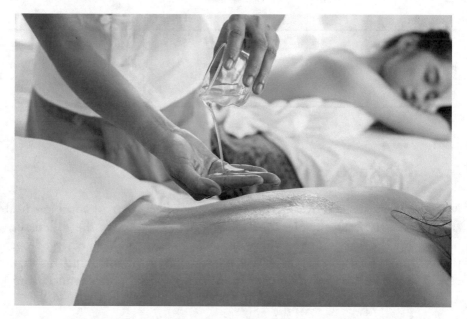

Fig. 4.1 Aromatherapy combines gentle massage techniques with the application of essential oils [*source* Free Images on Unsplash]

mood, quality of life and the intensity and bother of two symptoms most important to cancer patients.[16] A 2012 systematic review found no lasting effects but documented short-term effects of aromatherapy on depression, anxiety and overall well-being of cancer patients. Specifically, some clinical trials suggested symptomatic improvements such as enhanced well-being and sleep. Other trials reported short-term improvements in anxiety and depression scores and better pain control.[17] The current Cochrane review compared massage with and without aromatherapy and did not identify clinically relevant benefits for cancer patients (Fig. 4.1).[18]

The totality of this evidence indicates that aromatherapy massages might be experienced as agreeable and relaxing, however, they seem to convey few tangible health benefits to cancer patients.

---

[16] Wilcock A, Manderson C, Weller R, Walker G, Carr D, Carey AM, Broadhurst D, Mew J, Ernst E. Does aromatherapy massage benefit patients with cancer attending a specialist palliative care day centre? Palliat Med. 2004 May;18(4):287–90. https://doi.org/10.1191/0269216304pm895oa. PMID: 15198118.

[17] Boehm K, Büssing A, Ostermann T. Aromatherapy as an adjuvant treatment in cancer care—a descriptive systematic review. Afr J Tradit Complement Altern Med. 2012 Jul 1;9(4):503–18. https://doi.org/10.4314/ajtcam.v9i4.7. PMID: 23983386; PMCID: PMC3746639.

[18] Shin ES, Seo KH, Lee SH, Jang JE, Jung YM, Kim MJ, Yeon JY. Massage with or without aromatherapy for symptom relief in people with cancer. Cochrane Database Syst Rev. 2016 Jun 3;(6):CD009873. https://doi.org/10.1002/14651858.CD009873.pub3. PMID: 27258432.

Plausibility	👎
Effectiveness	👎
Safety	👍
Cost	👎
Risk/benefit balance	👎

Hot Stone Massage

Hot stone massage consists of placing the stones on the skin of the patient; alternatively, the therapist might apply a massage oil to the skin and manually move the stones along muscles or other anatomical structures. Therapists often employ Swedish massage techniques (see below) while the stones are in place or after they have been removed.

The localized heat and weight of the stones are supposed to warm and relax muscles, allowing the massage therapist to apply deeper pressure to those areas while causing less discomfort. Patients often experience hot stone massage as comforting and relaxing.

The therapeutic claims made for this treatment are similar to those made for massage therapy and include, for instance, an alleviation of anxiety, depression and musculoskeletal pain. There are, however, no rigorous studies testing the effectiveness of hot stone massage in palliative or supportive cancer care. Therefore, this therapy cannot be considered as an evidence-based cancer therapy.

Plausibility	👎
Effectiveness	👎
Safety	👍
Cost	👎
Risk/benefit balance	👎

Lymph-Drainage

Lymph-drainage is a gentle manual massage technique developed in the 1930s by Emil and Estrid Vodder. It consists of rhythmic manual movements along lymph vessels. This is said to further the flow of the lymph fluid through the lymphatic system towards the lymphnodes and into the blood circulation. Lymph-drainage is usually performed by massage therapists who have received special training in that method. A simplified version of the therapy can be taught to patients for regular self-treatments. The fear that lymph-drainage might spread cancer cells throughout the body has not been confirmed.

Lymph-drainage is best-studied as a treatment of lymphoedema, a condition that sometimes occurs after radical cancer surgery. A 2015 Cochrane review of 6 studies concluded that manual lymph-drainage (MLD) is safe and offers additional benefit to compression bandaging for swelling reduction. Findings were contradictory for function (range of motion), and inconclusive for quality of life. For symptoms such as pain and heaviness, most patients reported feeling better regardless of which treatment they received.[19]

In an RCT published in 2016, breast cancer patients with radical mastectomy received either physical exercise only (PE group, the control; $n = 500$) or self-MLD as well as exercise (MLD group; $n = 500$). In the PE group, patients started to undertake remedial exercises and progressive weight training after recovery from anaesthesia. In the MLD group, in addition to receiving the same treatments as in the PE group, the patients were trained to perform self-MLD on the surgical incision for 10 min/session, 3 sessions/day, beginning after suture removal and incision closure (10–30 days after the surgery). Compared to those in the PE group, patients in MLD group experienced significant improvements in scar contracture, shoulder abduction, and upper limb circumference. The authors concluded that *self-MLD, in combination with physical exercise, is beneficial for breast cancer patients in preventing postmastectomy scar formation, upper limb lymphedema, and shoulder joint dysfunction.*[20]

Finally, a 2018 study tested whether MLD or active exercise (AE) were associated with improvements in shoulder range of motion (ROM), wound complication and changes in the lymphatic parameters after breast cancer surgery, and whether these parameters had an association with lymphoedema

---

[19] Ezzo J, Manheimer E, McNeely ML, Howell DM, Weiss R, Johansson KI, Bao T, Bily L, Tuppo CM, Williams AF, Karadibak D. Manual lymphatic drainage for lymphedema following breast cancer treatment. Cochrane Database Syst Rev. 2015 May 21;(5):CD003475.

[20] Zhang L, Fan A, Yan J, He Y, Zhang H, Zhang H, Zhong Q, Liu F, Luo Q, Zhang L, Tang H, Xin M. Combining Manual Lymph Drainage with Physical Exercise after Modified Radical Mastectomy Effectively Prevents Upper Limb Lymphedema. Lymphat Res Biol. 2016 Jun;14(2):104–8. https://doi.org/10.1089/lrb.2015.0036. Epub 2016 Jan 29. PMID: 26824722.

formation in the long run. The researchers conducted a clinical trial with 106 women undergoing radical surgery for breast cancer and concluded that *MLD is as safe and effective as AE in rehabilitation after breast cancer surgery.*[21]

Plausibility	👍
Effectiveness	👍
Safety	👍
Cost	👎
Risk/benefit balance	👍

Collectively, these studies suggest that cancer patients can benefit from lymph-drainage in preventing and treating lymphoedema.

Reflexology

Reflexology is a manual technique where manual pressure is applied usually to the sole of the patient's foot. Reflexology is said to have its roots in ancient cultures. Its current popularity goes back to the US doctor William Fitzgerald (1872–1942) who thought to have discovered that the human body is divided into 10 zones each of which is represented on the sole of the foot.[22] Today, reflexologists have maps of the sole of the foot where all the body's organs are depicted. By massaging specific zones claimed to be connected to specific organs, reflexologists believe to positively influence the function of these organs. The assumptions that underpin reflexology lack plausibility.

Reflexology has nevertheless been submitted to clinical trials in several conditions, including diabetes, premenstrual syndrome, cancer patients, multiple sclerosis, symptomatic idiopathic detrusor over-activity and

---

[21] Oliveira MMF, Gurgel MSC, Amorim BJ, Ramos CD, Derchain S, Furlan-Santos N, Dos Santos CC, Sarian LO. Long-term effects of manual lymphatic drainage and active exercises on physical morbidities, lymphoscintigraphy parameters and lymphedema formation in patients operated due to breast cancer: A clinical trial. PLoS One. 2018 Jan 5;13(1):e0189176. https://doi.org/10.1371/jou rnal.pone.0189176. PMID: 29304140; PMCID: PMC5755747.

[22] http://www.reflexologyinstitute.com/reflex_fitzgerald.php.

dementia. However, most of these studies are of poor quality. A system-atic review concluded that *the best clinical evidence does not demonstrate convincingly reflexology to be an effective treatment for any medical condition.*[23]

Our own 2010 systematic review assessed the effectiveness of reflexology as a symptomatic treatment for breast cancer. One RCT and 3 non-randomized controlled clinical trials (CCTs) met our inclusion criteria. One large RCT showed significant differences in quality of life and mood when reflexology was compared with self-initiated support. Three CCTs tested reflexology compared with no treatment or simple rest. All of them suggested favourable effects of reflexology on pain, nausea, and vomiting. However, all had a high risk of bias. We concluded that, *collectively, the existing evidence does not convincingly show that reflexology is effective for breast cancer care.*[24]

A more recent study found that reflexology is more successful than atten-tion control in reducing cancer pain.[25] Unfortunately, this study did not control for placebo effects and other sources of bias.

In essence, this means that the evidence for reflexology as a palliative and supportive cancer therapy is not convincing. The treatment is undoubtedly experienced as agreeable by patients, but whether its effects go beyond the provision of some tender loving care (which is unquestionably important) seems debatable.

Plausibility	👎
Effectiveness	👎
Safety	👍
Cost	👎
Risk/benefit balance	👎

[23] Ernst E, Posadzki P, Lee MS. Reflexology: an update of a systematic review of randomised clinical trials. Maturitas. 2011 Feb;68(2):116–20. https://doi.org/10.1016/j.maturitas.2010.10.011. Epub 2010 Dec 15. PMID: 21111551.

[24] Kim JI, Lee MS, Kang JW, Choi DY, Ernst E. Reflexology for the symptomatic treatment of breast cancer: a systematic review. Integr Cancer Ther. 2010 Dec;9(4):326–30. https://doi.org/10.1177/153 4735410387423. PMID: 21106613.

[25] Sikorskii A, Niyogi PG, Victorson D, Tamkus D, Wyatt G. Symptom response analysis of a randomized controlled trial of reflexology for symptom management among women with advanced breast cancer. Support Care Cancer. 2020 Mar;28(3):1395–1404. https://doi.org/10.1007/s00520-019-04959-y. Epub 2019 Jul 2. PMID: 31267277; PMCID: PMC6939151.

Shiatsu

Shiatsu is a (mostly) manual therapy that was popularised by Japanese Toku-jiro Namikoshi (1905–2000). It developed out of the Chinese massage therapy, 'tui na' (see below). Shiatsu follows the principles of Traditional Chinese Medicine based on chi, meridians, yin and yang, etc. Shiatsu is claimed to stimulate the body's vital energy. These concepts lack scientific and biological plausibility.

The amount of pressure used during treatment can be considerable and Shiatsu is thus experienced by some patients as (mildly) painful. Shiatsu includes not just the pressure applied by the therapist at specific points but also awareness of body posture, breathing and exercise. One observational study found that 12–22% of patients reported 'negative effects' after shiatsu treatment,[26] and several case reports have associated Shiatsu with serious complications. e. g.[27]

Plausibility	👎
Effectiveness	👎
Safety	👍
Cost	👎
Risk/benefit balance	👎

There are no clinical trials of shiatsu as a palliative or supportive cancer therapy. Therefore, this treatment cannot be categorised as being evidence-based.

Swedish Massage

Swedish (or classical) massage consists of various manual techniques:

- effleurage (long smooth strokes),
- petrissage (kneading, rolling, and lifting),
- friction (wringing or small circular movements),
- tapotement (percussion),
- vibration (rocking and shaking movements).

---

[26] https://www.ncbi.nlm.nih.gov/pubmed/19398071.
[27] https://www.ncbi.nlm.nih.gov/pmc/articles/PMC1739324/.

In most European countries, Swedish massage (the name comes from the fact that the Swede, Per Henrik Ling was instrumental in developing the treatment) is considered to be part of conventional healthcare, while elsewhere it is usually viewed as a SCAM.

Several systematic reviews of clinical trials are currently available. They must, however, be interpreted with caution, since the types of massage therapy used are often not clearly differentiated. One overview identified 31 systematic reviews of massage for pain control, of which 21 were considered high-quality.[28] Two systematic reviews were focussed on cancer; they concluded that massage therapy shows promise in palliative and supportive cancer care suggesting that massage can alleviate a wide range of symptoms:

- pain,
- nausea,
- anxiety,
- depression,
- anger,
- stress,
- fatigue.

As the number and methodological quality of the primary studies are often low, definitive conclusions seem problematic.[29,30] Adverse effects of massage have been reported but are usually mild and infrequent.[31]

Swedish massage can thus be considered as a promising therapy for easing various symptoms of cancer patients.

Plausibility	👍
Effectiveness	👍

(continued)

[28] Miake-Lye I, Lee J, Lugar T, Taylor S, Shanman R, Beroes J, Shekelle P. Massage for Pain: An Evidence Map [Internet]. Washington (DC): Department of Veterans Affairs (US); 2016 Sep. PMID: 28211657.

[29] Ernst E. Massage therapy for cancer palliation and supportive care: a systematic review of randomised clinical trials. Support Care Cancer. 2009 Apr;17(4):333–7. https://doi.org/10.1007/s00520-008-0569-z. Epub 2009 Jan 13. PMID: 19148685.

[30] Lee MS, Lee EN, Ernst E. Massage therapy for breast cancer patients: a systematic review. Ann Oncol. 2011 Jun;22(6):1459–1461. https://doi.org/10.1093/annonc/mdr147. Epub 2011 May 4. PMID: 21543629.

[31] Ernst E. The safety of massage therapy. Rheumatology (Oxford). 2003 Sep;42(9):1101–6. https://doi.org/10.1093/rheumatology/keg306. Epub 2003 May 30. PMID: 12777645.

(continued)

Safety	👍
Cost	👎
Risk/benefit balance	👍/👎

Tui na

Tui na is a massage therapy that originates from Traditional Chinese Medicine. Many of the techniques used in tui na resemble those of a western massage like gliding, kneading, vibration, tapping, friction, pulling, rolling, pressing and shaking. Tui na involves a range of manipulations usually performed by the therapist's finger, hand, elbow, knee, or foot. They are applied to muscle or soft tissue at specific locations of the body.

Plausibility	👎
Effectiveness	👎
Safety	👍
Cost	👎
Risk/benefit balance	👎

The aim of tui na is to enhance the flow of the vital energy, chi, that is alleged to control our health. Proponents of the therapy recommend tui na for a range of conditions, including cancer. There are, however, no clinical studies to test whether tui na is effective for the problems experienced by cancer patients. Therefore, this treatment cannot be considered to be evidence-based.

4.3 Mind-Body Therapies

Mind-body therapies include a range of treatments aimed at influencing our health and well-being via the mind. They are commonly used SCAMs by cancer patients and are becoming increasingly popular. [32,33] Most mind-body therapies induce relaxation which, in turn, might be useful in palliative and supportive cancer care. One review, for instance, suggested that *mind-body therapies deal with common experiences that cause distress around cancer diagnosis, treatment, and survivorship including loss of control, uncertainty about the future, fears of recurrence, and a range of physical and psychological symptoms including depression, anxiety, insomnia, and fatigue.*[34]

In this chapter, I will discuss those mind-body therapies which are commonly used in palliative and supported cancer care.

Autogenic Training

Autogenic training can be described as a form of self-hypnosis. It consists of a set of very simple mental exercises using instructions directed at different parts of the body aimed at controlling perceptions, such as 'my right foot feels warm' or 'my left arm feels heavy'. Patients tend to report an intense sense of relaxation during and after a session of autogenic training.

The method can be taught in a series of lessons given by a qualified instructor. Once mastered, it should be practised regularly and does not normally require further supervision. Autogenic training is claimed to help with a range of (mostly stress-related) symptoms. A systematic review concluded that *autogenic training is effective for adults' stress management.*[35]

Only very few trials with cancer patients are currently available. An RCT examining the effects of a sleep management programme for 229 patients with different cancers, found that Progressive Muscular Relaxation (see below) and autogenic training were equally effective in enhancing various sleep parameters

[32] Wong CH, Sundberg T, Chung VC, Voiss P, Cramer H. Complementary medicine use in US adults with a history of colorectal cancer: a nationally representative survey. Support Care Cancer. 2021 Jan;29(1):271–278. https://doi.org/10.1007/s00520-020-05494-x. Epub 2020 May 1. PMID: 32358777.

[33] Daly WC, Han PKJ, Hayn M, Ryan ST, Hansen MH, Linscott JP, Trinh QD, Sammon JD. Meditative and mind-body practice among patients with genitourinary malignancy. Urol Oncol. 2021 Jan 8:S1078–1439(20)30426–9. https://doi.org/10.1016/j.urolonc.2020.09.011. Epub ahead of print. PMID: 33431327.

[34] Carlson LE. Distress Management Through Mind-Body Therapies in Oncology. J Natl Cancer Inst Monogr. 2017 Nov 1;2017(52). https://doi.org/10.1093/jncimonographs/lgx009. PMID: 29140490.

[35] Seo E, Kim S. [Effect of Autogenic Training for Stress Response: A Systematic Review and Meta-Analysis]. J Korean Acad Nurs. 2019 Aug;49(4):361–374. Korean. https://doi.org/10.4040/jkan.2019.49.4.361. PMID: 31477667.

and reducing the need for sleep medication.[36] Another RCT assessed the effects of autogenic training on the psychological status and immune system responses in 31 women after lumpectomy for breast cancer.[37] Women receiving autogenic training in addition to home visits experienced a significant improvement in depressive mood compared to women who only had the home visits.

Collectively, this evidence suggests that autogenic training is likely to be helpful in the palliative and supportive care of cancer patients.

Plausibility	👍
Effectiveness	👍
Safety	👍
Cost	👍
Risk/benefit balance	👍

Guided Imagery

Guided imagery (or visualisation) is a therapy where the patient is taught by a trained practitioner to evoke certain mental images, sounds, tastes, smells or other sensations associated with specific therapeutic aims in the hope to facilitate reaching these aims. It is often recommended as a symptomatic therapy for a range of conditions and said to alleviate symptoms such as pain, stress, anxiety, and low mood.

Our 2005 systematic review of imagery for cancer patients included 6 RCTs. Their methodological quality was mostly low. Three studies reported significant differences in measures of anxiety, comfort or emotional response to chemotherapy for patients who received imagery over the control groups. Two studies showed no differences between guided imagery and other interventions in any of the outcome measures. We concluded that *imagery, as a sole adjuvant cancer therapy may be psycho-supportive and increase comfort. There is*

---

[36] Simeit R, Deck R, Conta-Marx B. Sleep management training for cancer patients with insomnia. Support Care Cancer. 2004 Mar;12(3):176–83. https://doi.org/10.1007/s00520-004-0594-5. Epub 2004 Feb 4. PMID: 14760542.

[37] Hidderley M, Holt M. A pilot randomized trial assessing the effects of autogenic training in early-stage cancer patients in relation to psychological status and immune system responses. Eur J Oncol Nurs. 2004 Mar;8(1):61–5. https://doi.org/10.1016/j.ejon.2003.09.003. PMID: 15003745.

no compelling evidence to suggest positive effects on physical symptoms such as nausea and vomiting.[38]

This indicates that imagery is a promising option for alleviating certain symptoms during palliative and supportive cancer care.

Plausibility	👍
Effectiveness	👍
Safety	👍
Cost	👍
Risk/benefit balance	👍

Mindfulness

Mindfulness is a popular form of meditation which involves bringing one's attention to experiences occurring in the present moment while sitting silently and paying attention to thoughts, sounds, the sensations of breathing or parts of the body. There are several forms of mindfulness meditation; one of the most thoroughly researched is Mindfulness-Based Stress Reduction developed by Jon Kabat-Zinn (1944–). It uses a combination of mindfulness meditation, body awareness, and yoga to help people become more mindful.

There has been much research into mindfulness, and many studies are now available. However, the quality of these trials is often poor which is one reason why the evidence is less clear than one would hope. There are also many reviews of mindfulness for cancer patients. The most recent and rigorous of these reviews included 28 RCTs with a total of 3053 cancer patients. Mindfulness was associated with significant reductions in the severity of short-term and medium-term anxiety, but no reduction in long-term anxiety was observed. Mindfulness was furthermore associated with a reduction in the severity of depression in the short and the medium term, and it improved health-related quality of life in patients both in the short and the medium

---

[38] Roffe L, Schmidt K, Ernst E. A systematic review of guided imagery as an adjuvant cancer therapy. Psychooncology. 2005 Aug;14(8):607–17. https://doi.org/10.1002/pon.889. PMID: 15651053.

term. The authors concluded that mindfulness was *associated with reductions in anxiety and depression up to 6 months postintervention in adults with cancer.*[39]

These findings suggest that mindfulness can be an effective treatment for many cancer patients in palliative or supportive care.

Plausibility	👍
Effectiveness	👍
Safety	👍
Cost	👍
Risk/benefit balance	👍

Music Therapy

Music therapy is the use of music for therapeutic purposes, usually supervised by a trained therapist who has completed an approved music therapy programme. Several forms of music therapy exist. Patients might either passively listen to live or recorded music, or they actively participate in performing music. Therapists try to use all aspects of music, physical, emotional, mental, social, aesthetic, and spiritual.

A Cochrane review included 52 trials with a total of 3731 cancer patients. The results suggested that music interventions may have a beneficial effect on anxiety and a moderately strong, positive impact on depression. In addition, music therapy had a small to moderate treatment effect on fatigue and a large effect on patients' quality of life. The authors caution that, because of the poor quality of the included studies, these findings are less certain than one might hope. They concluded that *music interventions may have beneficial effects on anxiety, pain, fatigue and quality of life in people with cancer.*[40]

---

[39] Oberoi S, Yang J, Woodgate RL, Niraula S, Banerji S, Israels SJ, Altman G, Beattie S, Rabbani R, Askin N, Gupta A, Sung L, Abou-Setta AM, Zarychanski R. Association of Mindfulness-Based Interventions With Anxiety Severity in Adults With Cancer: A Systematic Review and Meta-analysis. JAMA Netw Open. 2020 Aug 3;3(8):e2012598. https://doi.org/10.1001/jamanetworkopen.2020.12598. PMID: 32766801; PMCID: PMC7414391.

[40] Bradt J, Dileo C, Magill L, Teague A. Music interventions for improving psychological and physical outcomes in cancer patients. Cochrane Database Syst Rev. 2016 Aug 15;(8):CD006911. https://doi.org/10.1002/14651858.CD006911.pub3. PMID: 27524661.

It seems likely from this evidence that music therapy might be useful to many cancer patients in palliative and supportive care.

Plausibility	👍
Effectiveness	👍
Safety	👍
Cost	👍
Risk/benefit balance	👍

Progressive Muscle Relaxation

Progressive muscle relaxation (PMR) was developed in the 1930s by the US physician Edmund Jacobson (1888–1983). The method has repeatedly been modified by others; consequently, several different variations of PMR currently exist. Patients are first taught to relax voluntary muscles. Once they have mastered this task, involuntary muscles follow automatically. Eventually, a 'relaxation response'[41] with deep relaxation of both the body and the mind is said to ensue.

The technique can be taught by initially actively tensing voluntary muscles and subsequently relaxing them. PMR allegedly causes a host of measurable physiological changes such as a reduction of stress hormones, a decrease of blood pressure, a slowing of heart frequency and respiratory rate. The method is used as a stress management technique and as an adjuvant treatment of a wide range of conditions associated with stress.

There have been numerous clinical trials of PMR as a therapy for cancer patients. A 2017 systematic review indicated that PMR might improve comfort and reduce the anxiety levels and side effects caused by chemotherapy. However, the quality of all the included studies was extremely low.[42] A 2020 systematic review found that that *PMR was a beneficial*

---

[41] https://en.wikipedia.org/wiki/The_Relaxation_Response.

[42] Pelekasis P, Matsouka I, Koumarianou A. Progressive muscle relaxation as a supportive intervention for cancer patients undergoing chemotherapy: A systematic review. Palliat Support Care. 2017 Aug;15(4):465–473. https://doi.org/10.1017/S1478951516000870. Epub 2016 Nov 28. PMID: 27890023.

approach preventing and alleviating chemotherapy-induced nausea and vomiting among cancer patients.[43]

Cancer patients suffering from such problems can thus be encouraged to try PMR.

Plausibility	👍
Effectiveness	👍
Safety	👍
Cost	👍
Risk/benefit balance	👍

Qigong

Qigong is a form of Traditional Chinese Medicine using meditation, exercise, deep breathing and other techniques with a view of strengthening the assumed life force 'qi'. There are several distinct forms of qigong which can be categorised into two main groups. Internal qigong refers to a physical and mental training method for the cultivation of oneself to achieve optimal health in both mind and body and is similar to tai (see below). External qigong refers to a treatment where qigong practitioners direct their qi-energy to the patient with the intention to clear qi-blockages or balance the flow of qi within that patient. External qigong has not been rigorously tested in the context of cancer; we therefore discuss here internal qigong only.

Several systematic reviews have become available:

- Our 2010 systematic review included 9 studies (4 were randomised trials and 5 were non-randomised studies). Eight of these trials tested internal qigong. The methodological quality of these studies varies greatly and was generally poor. All trials related to palliative and supportive cancer care. Two trials suggested effectiveness in prolonging life of cancer patients and

---

[43] Tian X, Tang RY, Xu LL, Xie W, Chen H, Pi YP, Chen WQ. Progressive muscle relaxation is effective in preventing and alleviating of chemotherapy-induced nausea and vomiting among cancer patients: a systematic review of six randomized controlled trials. Support Care Cancer. 2020 Sep;28(9):4051–4058. https://doi.org/10.1007/s00520-020-05481-2. Epub 2020 Apr 28. PMID: 32346796.

one failed to do so. We concluded that *the effectiveness of qigong in cancer care is not yet supported by the evidence from rigorous clinical trials.*[44]

- A 2012 systematic review included a total of 18 studies and arrived at a similar conclusion: *Due to high risk of bias and methodological problems in the majority of included studies, it is still too early to draw conclusive statements.*[45]

- Finally, a 2018 meta-analysis included 22 studies and concluded that *larger and methodologically sound trials with longer follow-up periods and appropriate comparison groups are needed before definitive conclusions can be drawn, and cancer- and symptom-specific recommendations can be made.*[46]

On balance, therefore, the evidence seems to be too weak for a positive recommendation of qigong in palliative and supportive cancer care.

Plausibility	👎
Effectiveness	👎
Safety	👍
Cost	👍
Risk/benefit balance	👎

Tai chi

Tai chi is an exercise therapy that involves meditative movements rooted in both Traditional Chinese Medicine and the martial arts. A number of different styles of tai chi have emerged. Tai chi can be taught in small classes in a quiet and relaxed atmosphere. Tai chi is seen as a life-long endeavour and

[44] Lee MS, Chen KW, Sancier KM, Ernst E. Qigong for cancer treatment: a systematic review of controlled clinical trials. Acta Oncol. 2007;46(6):717–22. https://doi.org/10.1080/02841860701261584. PMID: 17653892.

[45] Chan CL, Wang CW, Ho RT, Ng SM, Chan JS, Ziea ET, Wong VC. A systematic review of the effectiveness of qigong exercise in supportive cancer care. Support Care Cancer. 2012 Jun;20(6):1121–33. https://doi.org/10.1007/s00520-011-1378-3. Epub 2012 Jan 19. PMID: 22258414; PMCID: PMC3342492.

[46] Wayne PM, Lee MS, Novakowski J, Osypiuk K, Ligibel J, Carlson LE, Song R. Tai Chi and Qigong for cancer-related symptoms and quality of life: a systematic review and meta-analysis. J Cancer Surviv. 2018 Apr;12(2):256–267. https://doi.org/10.1007/s11764-017-0665-5. Epub 2017 Dec 8. PMID: 29222705; PMCID: PMC5958892.

regular practice of 2–3 sessions of about 30 min per week are recommended for optimal effects.

The effectiveness of tai chi has recently been the subject of many studies. Several systematic reviews have become available; yet, many of them are somewhat uncritical.

- Based on the 4 studies available in 2007, we concluded that the evidence is not convincing enough to suggest that tai chi is an effective supportive treatment for cancer.[47]
- In 2010, we published a further systematic review which showed that all non-randomised studies yielded positive findings while randomised trials failed to do so.[48]
- A 2018 systematic review included 6 RCTs and found that Tai Chi for more than 8 weeks has short-term ameliorative effects on cancer-related fatigue, especially among patients with breast and lung cancer. Its beneficial effects are superior to physical exercise and psychological support. It remains unclear whether there are long-term benefits, and further study is needed.[49]
- Finally, a systematic review of 2019 included 22 RCTs and concluded that *there is low-level evidence suggesting that Tai Chi improves physical and mental dimensions of quality of life and sleep. There is moderate-level evidence suggesting Tai Chi reduces levels of cortisol and cancer-related fatigue and improves limb function.*[50]

These reviews demonstrate that, during the last decade, the evidence for tai chi has become more numerous and more compelling. Today, it seems strong enough to categorise tai chi as an evidence-based treatment for cancer palliation and supportive care.

---

[47] Lee MS, Pittler MH, Ernst E. Is Tai Chi an effective adjunct in cancer care? A systematic review of controlled clinical trials. Support Care Cancer. 2007 Jun;15(6):597–601. https://doi.org/10.1007/s00520-007-0221-3. Epub 2007 Feb 21. PMID: 17318592.

[48] Lee MS, Choi TY, Ernst E. Tai chi for breast cancer patients: a systematic review. Breast Cancer Res Treat. 2010 Apr;120(2):309–16. https://doi.org/10.1007/s10549-010-0741-2. Epub 2010 Feb 2. PMID: 20127280.

[49] Song S, Yu J, Ruan Y, Liu X, Xiu L, Yue X. Ameliorative effects of Tai Chi on cancer-related fatigue: a meta-analysis of randomized controlled trials. Support Care Cancer. 2018 Jul;26(7):2091–2102. https://doi.org/10.1007/s00520-018-4136-y. Epub 2018 Mar 21. PMID: 29564620.

[50] Ni X, Chan RJ, Yates P, Hu W, Huang X, Lou Y. The effects of Tai Chi on quality of life of cancer survivors: a systematic review and meta-analysis. Support Care Cancer. 2019 Oct;27(10):3701–3716. https://doi.org/10.1007/s00520-019-04911-0. Epub 2019 Jun 24. PMID: 31236699.

Plausibility	👆
Effectiveness	👍
Safety	👍
Cost	👍
Risk/benefit balance	👍

4.4   Herbal Remedies

Many herbal remedies are being promoted as treatments that help cancer patients in reducing their symptoms and thus improving their quality of life. But which are truly effective? Here I will discuss those that are popular and for which at least a minimal amount of evidence is currently available.

Aloe vera

Aloe vera is a plant that belongs to the *Liliaceae* family. There are many aloe species; for medicinal purposes, *Aloe barbadensis* is the most commonly used. It contains more than 200 different pharmacologically active substances, including minerals and vitamins, various polysaccharides and phenolic chemicals, notably anthraquinones[51]. They are said to have immunomodulatory, anti-viral, anti-bacterial, anti-inflammatory, anti-arthritic, anti-cancer, anti-diabetic and wound-healing properties.

Two fundamentally different types of Aloe vera preparations exist:

- Aloe vera gel is used topically and is made of the mucillaginous centre of the plant's leaf.
- Oral aloe vera preparations are made from the plant's peripheral bundle sheath cells.

---

[51] Radha MH, Laxmipriya NP. Evaluation of biological properties and clinical effectiveness of Aloe vera: A systematic review. J Tradit Complement Med. 2014 Dec 23;5(1):21–6. https://doi.org/10.1016/j.jtcme.2014.10.006. PMID: 26151005; PMCID: PMC4488101.

The gel preparations are often recommended for treating the skin problems of cancer patients. A 2005 systematic review concluded that *there is no evidence from clinical trials to suggest that topical Aloe vera is effective in preventing or minimising radiation-induced skin reactions in cancer patients.*[52] A 2019 systematic review, however, was less pessimistic and suggested that *Aloe vera may be effective … for acute radiation proctitis.*[53] No serious adverse effects are on record.

In essence, this means that aloe vera gel is supported by encouraging albeit not compelling evidence as a possible treatment for radiation injury in cancer patients.

Plausibility	👍
Effectiveness	👎
Safety	👍
Cost	👍
Risk/benefit balance	👎

Calendula

Calendula is a topical treatment derived from *Calendula officinalis*, a plant of the marigold family, which contains numerous polyphenolic antioxidants. Calendula has been studied in both the laboratory and clinical setting for treating and preventing radiation-induced skin irritations. Despite some preclinical evidence supporting calendula's mechanism of action in preventing radiation-induced skin toxicity, the results of clinical studies are contradictory and therefore not convincing.

A 2015 systematic review concluded that *Calendula appears to be a safe topical therapy in the treatment and prevention of radiation-induced skin toxicity, however*

---

[52] Richardson J, Smith JE, McIntyre M, Thomas R, Pilkington K. Aloe vera for preventing radiation-induced skin reactions: a systematic literature review. Clin Oncol (R Coll Radiol). 2005 Sep;17(6):478–84. https://doi.org/10.1016/j.clon.2005.04.013. PMID: 16149293.

[53] Farrugia CE, Burke ES, Haley ME, Bedi KT, Gandhi MA. The use of aloe vera in cancer radiation: An updated comprehensive review. Complement Ther Clin Pract. 2019 May;35:126–130. https://doi.org/10.1016/j.ctcp.2019.01.013. Epub 2019 Jan 31. PMID: 31003648.

the evidence for its use remains weak. Its efficacy compared to other therapies is, however, still in question given the conflicting data reported in previous studies.[54]

Plausibility	👍
Effectiveness	🤚
Safety	👍
Cost	👍
Risk/benefit balance	🤚

Cannabis

Cannabis (*Cannabis sativa L.*) has a long history of medicinal use (Sect. 3.1). Cannabinoids that have been approved for medical purposes contain delta-9-tetrahydrocannabinol (THC). While they were derived from a plant, they do not contain the full spectrum of its ingredients. Therefore, they cannot be categorised as herbal remedies.

Cannabinoids may be a useful therapeutic option for people with chemotherapy-induced nausea and vomiting or pain. Several systematic reviews are available:

- A 2015 Cochrane review included 23 RCTs. Its findings showed that *cannabis-based medications may be useful for treating refractory chemotherapy-induced nausea and vomiting. However, methodological limitations of the trials limit the conclusions.*[55]
- A 2020 review concluded that *good preclinical animal data and a large body of observational evidence point to the potential efficacy of cannabinoids for*

---

[54] Kodiyan J, Amber KT. A Review of the Use of Topical Calendula in the Prevention and Treatment of Radiotherapy-Induced Skin Reactions. Antioxidants (Basel). 2015 Apr 23;4(2):293–303. https://doi.org/10.3390/antiox4020293. PMID: 26783706; PMCID: PMC4665477.

[55] Smith LA, Azariah F, Lavender VT, Stoner NS, Bettiol S. Cannabinoids for nausea and vomiting in adults with cancer receiving chemotherapy. Cochrane Database Syst Rev. 2015 Nov 12;2015(11):CD009464. https://doi.org/10.1002/14651858.CD009464.pub2. PMID: 26561338; PMCID: PMC6931414.

cancer pain management. However, there are relatively weak data pointing to clinical efficacy from clinical trial data to date.[56]

- A 2020 systematic review included 8 studies with cancer patients undergoing radiotherapy (RT). The findings suggested that *the use of cannabinoids may calm anxious patients about to start RT, reduce nausea and vomiting consistent with the contemporary standard of care, reduce the symptoms of relapse for patients with glioma, and provide symptom relief after head and neck RT.*[57]

Thus there is reasonably sound evidence to suggest that cannabinoid medications might be worth a try for patients who did not respond to conventional therapies.

Plausibility	👍
Effectiveness	👍
Safety	👎
Cost	👎
Risk/benefit balance	👍

Chamomile

Chamomile is a popular herbal remedy that is being promoted against a range of conditions. Chamomile mouthwash is recommended against radiation-induced mucositis, a common problem of cancer patients after radiotherapy. The only RCT testing its effectiveness, however, failed to generate positive results. Its authors concluded that *this clinical trial did not support the pre-study hypothesis that chamomile could decrease 5-FU-induced stomatitis.*[58]

Therefore chamomile cannot be regarded as an evidence-based option during palliative or supportive cancer care.

---

[56] Meng H, Dai T, Hanlon JG, Downar J, Alibhai SMH, Clarke H. Cannabis and cannabinoids in cancer pain management. Curr Opin Support Palliat Care. 2020 Jun;14(2):87–93. https://doi.org/10.1097/SPC.0000000000000493. PMID: 32332209.

[57] Rosewall T, Feuz C, Bayley A. Cannabis and Radiation Therapy: A Scoping Review of Human Clinical Trials. J Med Imaging Radiat Sci. 2020 Jun;51(2):342–349. https://doi.org/10.1016/j.jmir.2020.01.007. Epub 2020 Apr 3. PMID: 32249134.

[58] Fidler P, Loprinzi CL, O'Fallon JR, Leitch JM, Lee JK, Hayes DL, Novotny P, Clemens-Schutjer D, Bartel J, Michalak JC. Prospective evaluation of a chamomile mouthwash for prevention of 5-FU-induced oral mucositis. Cancer. 1996 Feb 1;77(3):522–5. https://doi.org/10.1002/(SICI)1097-0142(19960201)77:3<522::AID-CNCR14>3.0.CO;2-6.

Plausibility	👍
Effectiveness	👎
Safety	👍
Cost	👍
Risk/benefit balance	👎

Chinese Herbal Mixtures

Chinese herbal medicine has a long history and is still being used in China alongside conventional medicine. There are thousands of plants used medicinally, and in Chinese herbal medicine, they are typically combined in mixtures that contain a multitude of different plants. The ancient Chinese literature recorded more than 100 000 medicinal recipes some of which also contain non-botanical ingredients such as minerals and animal parts. Generalisations regarding the effectiveness or safety across all Chinese herbal medicines are therefore impossible.

Most of the research into Chinese herbal medicines is published in Chinese, and there are several reasons to be sceptical about its reliability; fraud seems to be rife and Chinese researchers publish only positive results.[59]

A 2016 systematic review included 14 RCTs. Compared with conventional intervention alone, combined Chinese herbal mixtures (CHM) together with conventional treatments significantly reduced pain. Six trials comparing CHM with conventional medications demonstrated similar effect in reducing constipation. One RCT showed significant positive effect of CHM plus chemotherapy for managing fatigue. The additional use of CHM to chemotherapy did not improve anorexia when compared to chemotherapy alone.[60]

---

[59] Tang JL, Zhan SY, Ernst E. Review of randomised controlled trials of traditional Chinese medicine. BMJ. 1999 Jul 17;319(7203):160–1. https://doi.org/10.1136/bmj.319.7203.160. PMID: 10406751; PMCID: PMC28166.

[60] Chung VC, Wu X, Lu P, Hui EP, Zhang Y, Zhang AL, Lau AY, Zhao J, Fan M, Ziea ET, Ng BF, Wong SY, Wu JC. Chinese Herbal Medicine for Symptom Management in Cancer Palliative Care: Systematic Review And Meta-analysis. Medicine (Baltimore). 2016 Feb;95(7):e2793. https://doi.org/10.1097/MD.0000000000002793. Erratum in: Medicine (Baltimore). 2016 May 20;95(20):e6650. PMID: 26886628; PMCID: PMC4998628.

Due to the many problems with CHM, it seems unjustified to recommend them to cancer patients.

Plausibility	
Effectiveness	
Safety	
Cost	
Risk/benefit balance	

Curcumin

Curcumin is an ingredient of turmeric (*Curcuma longa*) which belongs to the ginger family, *Zingiberaceae*, and is native to southern Asia. Turmeric has been used extensively in Ayurvedic medicine and has a variety of pharmacologic properties including antioxidant, analgesic, anti-inflammatory, and antiseptic activities. Therefore, turmeric has potential in several different areas. Yet, there are important open questions; one recent review, for instance, cautioned because of *its extremely low oral bioavailability hampers its application as therapeutic agent.*[61]

A 2020 systematic review included 22 clinical trials and suggested that curcumin can reduce side effects during cancer palliation such as skin irritation and side effects of chemotherapy. Curcumin intake during radiation therapy for breast cancer patients improved treatment outcomes, prevented skin symptoms, reduced pain and improved their quality of life.[62] Another review summarised preliminary results indicating that curcumin may serve as an options for preventing oral mucositis in cancer patients following radiotherapy.[63]

---

[61] Liu W, Zhai Y, Heng X, Che FY, Chen W, Sun D, Zhai G. Oral bioavailability of curcumin: problems and advancements. J Drug Target. 2016 Sep;24(8):694–702. https://doi.org/10.3109/106 1186X.2016.1157883. Epub 2016 Mar 17. PMID: 26942997.

[62] Mansouri K, Rasoulpoor S, Daneshkhah A, Abolfathi S, Salari N, Mohammadi M, Rasoulpoor S, Shabani S. Clinical effects of curcumin in enhancing cancer therapy: A systematic review. BMC Cancer. 2020 Aug 24;20(1):791. https://doi.org/10.1186/s12885-020-07256-8. PMID: 32838749; PMCID: PMC7446227.

[63] Yu YY, Deng JL, Jin XR, Zhang ZZ, Zhang XH, Zhou X. Effects of 9 oral care solutions on the prevention of oral mucositis: a network meta-analysis of randomized controlled trials.

Despite the current hype about curcumin, its effectiveness as a palliative or supportive cancer treatment remains unproven.

Plausibility	👍
Effectiveness	👎
Safety	👍
Cost	👍
Risk/benefit balance	👎

Ginger

Ginger (*Zingiber officinale*) is a perennial plant native to southern Asia. It has been traditionally used for a range of conditions, including the treatment of nausea.

A systematic review published in 2013 included 7 studies of oral ginger intake for chemotherapy-induced nausea and vomiting (CINV). Its authors concluded that studies were mixed in their support of ginger as an anti-CINV treatment in patients receiving chemotherapy, with three demonstrating a positive effect, two in favour but with caveats, and two showing no effect on measures of CINV.[64] By 2019, there were 10 studies that could be included in a meta-analysis. The authors were then able to show that *Ginger displayed significant efficacy with regard to controlling CINV in the experimental groups.*[65]

The evidence is thus encouraging, and ginger seems to be a reasonable option that might be worth trying for patients suffering from CINV who do not respond to conventional treatments.

Medicine (Baltimore). 2020 Apr;99(16):e19661. https://doi.org/10.1097/MD.0000000000019661. PMID: 32311938; PMCID: PMC7220734.

[64] Marx WM, Teleni L, McCarthy AL, Vitetta L, McKavanagh D, Thomson D, Isenring E. Ginger (Zingiber officinale) and chemotherapy-induced nausea and vomiting: a systematic literature review. Nutr Rev. 2013 Apr;71(4):245–54. https://doi.org/10.1111/nure.12016. Epub 2013 Mar 13. PMID: 23550785.

[65] Chang WP, Peng YX. Does the Oral Administration of Ginger Reduce Chemotherapy-Induced Nausea and Vomiting?: A Meta-analysis of 10 Randomized Controlled Trials. Cancer Nurs. 2019 Nov/Dec;42(6):E14–E23. https://doi.org/10.1097/NCC.0000000000000648. PMID: 30299420.

Plausibility	👍
Effectiveness	👍
Safety	👍
Cost	👍
Risk/benefit balance	👍

Ginseng

American ginseng (*Panax quinquefolius, Panacis quinquefolis*) and Asian ginseng (Panax ginseng) are often recommended against cancer-related fatigue.

Several studies have tested their effectiveness for this purpose.[66,67,68] Their methodological quality is mostly poor, and their findings are contradictory. On balance, the evidence is therefore not convincing.

Plausibility	👍
Effectiveness	🤚
Safety	👍
Cost	👍
Risk/benefit balance	🤚

[66] Barton DL, Liu H, Dakhil SR, Linquist B, Sloan JA, Nichols CR, McGinn TW, Stella PJ, Seeger GR, Sood A, Loprinzi CL. Wisconsin Ginseng (Panax quinquefolius) to improve cancer-related fatigue: a randomized, double-blind trial, N07C2. J Natl Cancer Inst. 2013 Aug 21;105(16):1230–8. https://doi.org/10.1093/jnci/djt181. Epub 2013 Jul 13. PMID: 23853057; PMCID: PMC3888141.

[67] Guglielmo M, Di Pede P, Alfieri S, Bergamini C, Platini F, Ripamonti CI, Orlandi E, Iacovelli NA, Licitra L, Maddalo M, Bossi P. A randomized, double-blind, placebo controlled, phase II study to evaluate the efficacy of ginseng in reducing fatigue in patients treated for head and neck cancer. J Cancer Res Clin Oncol. 2020 Oct;146(10):2479–2487. https://doi.org/10.1007/s00432-020-033 00-z. Epub 2020 Jul 2. PMID: 32617701.

[68] Arring NM, Millstine D, Marks LA, Nail LM. Ginseng as a Treatment for Fatigue: A Systematic Review. J Altern Complement Med. 2018 Jul;24(7):624–633. https://doi.org/10.1089/acm.2017. 0361. Epub 2018 Apr 6. PMID: 29624410.

Guarana

Guarana (*Paullinia cupana*) is a climbing plant of the family *Sapindaceae*, native to the Amazon basin and commonly used in Brazil. As a dietary supplement, it is used mostly as a stimulant. The plant contains about twice the concentration of caffeine found in coffee seeds and is thus being used in many energy drinks. It is thus unsurprising that guarana is often recommended also against cancer-related fatigue.

Several trials have tested its effectiveness and suggested that it is helpful for this purpose. One such study, for instance, concluded that *Guarana is an effective, inexpensive, and nontoxic alternative for the short-term treatment of fatigue in breast cancer patients receiving systemic chemotherapy.*[69]

The collective evidence indicates that guarana is a herbal supplement or drink that may well be worth trying for patients suffering from cancer-related fatigue.

Plausibility	👍
Effectiveness	👍
Safety	✋
Cost	👍
Risk/benefit balance	👍

Individualised Herbalism

Traditional herbalists come in numerous guises depending on what tradition they belong to: Chinese herbalists, traditional European herbalists, Ayurvedic practitioners, Kampo practitioners, Tibetan herbalists, etc. Their treatments are fundamentally different from those of rational herbal medicine: they are

---

69 de Oliveira Campos MP, Riechelmann R, Martins LC, Hassan BJ, Casa FB, Del Giglio A. Guarana (Paullinia cupana) improves fatigue in breast cancer patients undergoing systemic chemotherapy. J Altern Complement Med. 2011 Jun;17(6):505–12. https://doi.org/10.1089/acm.2010.0571. Epub 2011 May 25. PMID: 21612429.

not primarily focussed on the disease the patient is suffering from, but are individualised according to the specific characteristics of each patient.

Globally, traditional herbal therapy is by far the most common form of herbal medicine. Traditional herbalists frequently do not recognise the diagnostic categories of conventional medicine, but employ their very own (usually unvalidated) diagnostic methods (e. g. 'tongue and pulse diagnoses' used by Chinese herbalists). They are thus inclined to treat any condition, including cancer.

Contrary to what many traditional herbalists claim, the efficacy of the individualised herbal approach can be tested in rigorous trials. The totality of such studies yield no good evidence to show that it is effective. The only systematic review of these studies concluded that *there is no convincing evidence to support the use of individualised herbal medicine in any indication.*[70]

The risk of harm through individualised herbal mixtures can be considerable: the more ingredients, the higher the likelihood of toxicity, or interactions with prescription drugs taken by cancer patients.

Essentially, this means that there is no good evidence to demonstrate that individualised herbal treatments are of benefit to cancer patients.

Plausibility	👎
Effectiveness	👎
Safety	👎
Cost	👎
Risk/benefit balance	👎

Mistletoe

Mistletoe (*Viscum album*) is a semi-parasitic plant that grows on host trees such as oak, elm, pine and apple. Its use as a caner treatment goes back to Rudolf Steiner (1861–1925) and his anthroposophical medicine. Together with the medical doctor Ita Wegman (1876–1943), Steiner developed his mistletoe preparation, 'Iscador' (Weleda). Iscador is a fermented mistletoe

[70] Guo R, Canter PH, Ernst E. A systematic review of randomised clinical trials of individualised herbal medicine in any indication. Postgrad Med J. 2007 Oct;83(984):633–7. https://doi.org/10.1136/pgmj.2007.060202. PMID: 17916871; PMCID: PMC2600130.

extract and still the most widely used mistletoe product. Today, many other mistletoe preparations are available from various other manufacturers. The claim is that firstly they cure cancer (Sect. 3.1) and secondly they improve the quality of life of cancer patients receiving palliative or supportive care.

Numerous reviews of mistletoe have been published. Many are authored by ardent advocates of anthroposophic medicine and lack rigour or objectivity. A high-quality systematic review by a team of German oncologists included 28 publications with a total of 2639 patients. Mistletoe was used in bladder cancer, breast cancer, other gynaecological cancers (cervical cancer, corpus uteri cancer, and ovarian cancer), colorectal cancer, other gastrointestinal cancer (gastric cancer and pancreatic cancer), glioma, head and neck cancer, lung cancer, melanoma and osteosarcoma. In nearly all studies, mistletoe was added to a conventional therapy. Regarding quality of life, 17 trials reported results. Studies with better methodological quality showed less or no effects on quality of life. The authors concluded that *with respect to quality of life or reduction of treatment-associated side effects, a thorough review of the literature does not provide any indication to prescribe mistletoe to patients.*[71]

Contrary to statements by many SCAM proponents, mistletoe does not seem to be an effective therapy for improving the quality of life of cancer patients.

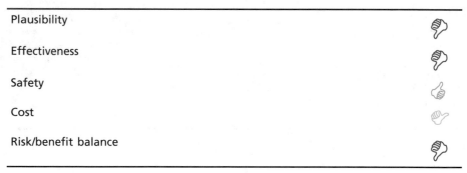

Plausibility	👎
Effectiveness	👎
Safety	👍
Cost	🤙
Risk/benefit balance	👎

4.5   Non-herbal Supplements

Dietary supplements are products taken orally as a pill, capsule, tablet, or liquid that are intended to supplement consumers' diet and are considered to

[71] Freuding M, Keinki C, Kutschan S, Micke O, Buentzel J, Huebner J. Mistletoe in oncological treatment: a systematic review : Part 2: quality of life and toxicity of cancer treatment. J Cancer Res Clin Oncol. 2019 Apr;145(4):927–939. https://doi.org/10.1007/s00432-018-02838-3. Epub 2019 Jan 23. PMID: 30673872.

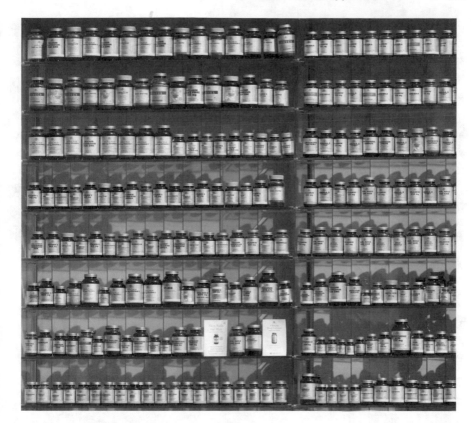

Fig. 4.2 The range of commercially available dietary supplements is vast [*source* Free Images on Unsplash]

be neither food nor medicine. They can contain herbal ingredients (Sect. 4.4), minerals, vitamins, fibre, amino acids, animal products. Globally, there are well over 100 000 different dietary supplements and the annual turnover currently exceeds US$ 60 billion. Many herbal (Sect. 4.4) and non-herbal supplements, the subject of this chapter, are being promoted to improve the life of cancer patients (Fig. 4.2).

Coenzyme Q10

Coenzyme Q10 (CoQ10) is a molecule that is produced in our bodies to partake in several important functions. It is also being marketed as a dietary supplement and is often promoted as a supportive treatment for cancer.

Our systematic review included 6 studies and suggested that CoQ10 might provide some protection against cardiotoxicity or liver toxicity during cancer treatment. However, because of the poor quality of the trials, the evidence was weak. We concluded that *suggestions that CoQ10 might reduce the toxicity of cancer treatments have not been tested by rigorous trials. Further investigations are necessary to determine whether CoQ10 can improve the tolerability of cancer treatments.*[72] Coenzyme Q10 can interact with prescribed medications and can cause adverse effects, including liver damage, nausea and headache. Preliminary evidence suggests that coenzyme Q10, both before and during breast cancer treatment, might be associated with an increased risk of recurrence and death.[73]

On balance, therefore, it seems questionable whether dietary supplements with CoQ10 generate more good than harm for cancer patients.

Plausibility	👎
Effectiveness	👎
Safety	👎
Cost	👎
Risk/benefit balance	👎

Fish Oil

Fish oil (omega-3) preparations are amongst the best-researched dietary supplements. Initial research demonstrated that the regular consumption of fish oil had a multitude of cardiovascular and anti-inflammatory effects. This led to the promotion of fish oil supplements for a wide range of conditions. Meanwhile, many of these early findings have been overturned by more rigorous studies,[74] and the enthusiasm for fish oil supplements has somewhat waned.

---

[72] Roffe L, Schmidt K, Ernst E. Efficacy of coenzyme Q10 for improved tolerability of cancer treatments: a systematic review. J Clin Oncol. 2004 Nov 1;22(21):4418–24. https://doi.org/10.1200/JCO.2004.02.034. PMID: 15514384.

[73] Ambrosone CB, Zirpoli GR, Hutson AD, McCann WE, McCann SE, Barlow WE, Kelly KM, Cannioto R, Sucheston-Campbell LE, Hershman DL, Unger JM, Moore HCF, Stewart JA, Isaacs C, Hobday TJ, Salim M, Hortobagyi GN, Gralow JR, Budd GT, Albain KS. Dietary Supplement Use During Chemotherapy and Survival Outcomes of Patients With Breast Cancer Enrolled in a Cooperative Group Clinical Trial (SWOG S0221). J Clin Oncol. 2020 Mar 10;38(8):804–814. https://doi.org/10.1200/JCO.19.01203. Epub 2019 Dec 19. PMID: 31855498; PMCID: PMC7062457.

[74] Abdelhamid AS, Brown TJ, Brainard JS, Biswas P, Thorpe GC, Moore HJ, Deane KH, AlAbdulghafoor FK, Summerbell CD, Worthington HV, Song F, Hooper L. Omega-3 fatty acids for the primary and secondary prevention of cardiovascular disease. Cochrane Database Syst Rev. 2018

As to cancer, the evidence is mixed:

- A 2012 systematic review of 38 studies concluded that *there is not enough evidence to support a net benefit of n-3-FA in cachexia in advanced cancer.*[75]
- A 2006 systematic review suggested that fish oil supplements for cancer patients had *inconsistent positive effects on survival and quality of life.*[76]
- A 2015 systematic review found that, in cancer patients, fish oil intake *can reduce inflammation and has the potential to modulate nutritional status/body composition.*[77]

Thus the evidence that omega-3 supplements are helpful during cancer palliative or supportive treatment is weak and inconclusive.

Plausibility	👎
Effectiveness	👎
Safety	👍
Cost	👍
Risk/benefit balance	👎

Melatonin

Melatonin is a hormone which is secreted by the pineal gland during night-time acting as a physiological regulator (Sect. 3.4). It is produced from tryptophan which is converted to serotonin and then enzymatically converted to melatonin. Dietary supplements or medications containing synthetically produced melatonin are available in most countries. Melatonin is used to

Jul 18;7(7):CD003177. https://doi.org/10.1002/14651858.CD003177.pub3. Update in: Cochrane Database Syst Rev. 2018 Nov 30;11:CD003177. PMID: 30019766; PMCID: PMC6513557.

75 Ries A, Trottenberg P, Elsner F, Stiel S, Haugen D, Kaasa S, Radbruch L. A systematic review on the role of fish oil for the treatment of cachexia in advanced cancer: an EPCRC cachexia guidelines project. Palliat Med. 2012 Jun;26(4):294–304. https://doi.org/10.1177/0269216311418709. Epub 2011 Aug 24. PMID: 21865295.

76 Elia M, Van Bokhorst-de van der Schueren MA, Garvey J, Goedhart A, Lundholm K, Nitenberg G, Stratton RJ. Enteral (oral or tube administration) nutritional support and eicosapentaenoic acid in patients with cancer: a systematic review. Int J Oncol. 2006 Jan;28(1):5–23. https://doi.org/10.3892/ijo.28.1.5. PMID: 16327975.

77 Pappalardo G, Almeida A, Ravasco P. Eicosapentaenoic acid in cancer improves body composition and modulates metabolism. Nutrition. 2015 Apr;31(4):549–55. https://doi.org/10.1016/j.nut.2014.12.002. Epub 2014 Dec 12. PMID: 25770317.

treat a range of problems that occur during palliative and supportive cancer care.

A 2014 systematic review found that, in cancer patients, melatonin significantly reduced asthenia, leukopenia, nausea and vomiting, hypotension, and thrombocytopenia.[78] More recent RCTs have added to this evidence:

- One study showed that, in breast cancer patients, melatonin reduces the adverse effects of chemotherapy on cognitive function, sleep quality and depressive symptoms.[79]
- Another trial found that the administration of melatonin with conventional treatment reduced severe radiation-induced oral mucositis development.[80]
- One study demonstrated that adjuvant melatonin delayed the onset of oral mucositis, which enabled uninterrupted cancer treatment and reduced the amount of morphine used for pain treatment.[81]
- Another trial showed that melatonin significantly reduced radiation dermatitis compared to placebo.[82]
- A further study found that melatonin significantly improved sleep efficiency after sleep onset after breast cancer surgery.[83]

In essence, the collective evidence seems to indicate that melatonin shows promise but more studies are needed to be sure.

---

[78] Seely D, Wu P, Fritz H, Kennedy DA, Tsui T, Seely AJ, Mills E. Melatonin as adjuvant cancer care with and without chemotherapy: a systematic review and meta-analysis of randomized trials. Integr Cancer Ther. 2012 Dec;11(4):293–303. https://doi.org/10.1177/1534735411425484. Epub 2011 Oct 21. PMID: 22019490.

[79] Palmer ACS, Zortea M, Souza A, Santos V, Biazús JV, Torres ILS, Fregni F, Caumo W. Clinical impact of melatonin on breast cancer patients undergoing chemotherapy; effects on cognition, sleep and depressive symptoms: A randomized, double-blind, placebo-controlled trial. PLoS One. 2020 Apr 17;15(4):e0231379. https://doi.org/10.1371/journal.pone.0231379. PMID: 32302347; PMCID: PMC7164654.

[80] Elsabagh HH, Moussa E, Mahmoud SA, Elsaka RO, Abdelrahman H. Efficacy of Melatonin in prevention of radiation-induced oral mucositis: A randomized clinical trial. Oral Dis. 2020 Apr;26(3):566–572. https://doi.org/10.1111/odi.13265. Epub 2020 Jan 15. PMID: 31869853.

[81] Onseng K, Johns NP, Khuayjarernpanishk T, Subongkot S, Priprem A, Hurst C, Johns J. Beneficial Effects of Adjuvant Melatonin in Minimizing Oral Mucositis Complications in Head and Neck Cancer Patients Receiving Concurrent Chemoradiation. J Altern Complement Med. 2017 Dec;23(12):957–963. https://doi.org/10.1089/acm.2017.0081. Epub 2017 Jun 28. PMID: 28657801.

[82] Ben-David MA, Elkayam R, Gelernter I, Pfeffer RM. Melatonin for Prevention of Breast Radiation Dermatitis: A Phase II, Prospective, Double-Blind Randomized Trial. Isr Med Assoc J. 2016 Mar-Apr;18(3–4):188–92. PMID: 27228641.

[83] Madsen MT, Hansen MV, Andersen LT, Hageman I, Rasmussen LS, Bokmand S, Rosenberg J, Gögenur I. Effect of Melatonin on Sleep in the Perioperative Period after Breast Cancer Surgery: A Randomized, Double-Blind, Placebo-Controlled Trial. J Clin Sleep Med. 2016 Feb;12(2):225–33. https://doi.org/10.5664/jcsm.5490. PMID: 26414973; PMCID: PMC4751412.

Plausibility	👍
Effectiveness	👍/👎
Safety	👍
Cost	👍
Risk/benefit balance	👍/👎

Probiotics

Probiotics are live microorganisms that are said to confer numerous health benefits (Sect. 3.4). Positive effects of probiotics on the systemic immune system have been demonstrated. Cancer patients tend to be immune-compromised and therefore need protection from infections.

A 2010 placebo-controlled RCT evaluated the effects of the enteral administration of the probiotic *Bifidobacterium breve* on its ability to prevent infections in cancer patients who had to receive chemotherapy. The frequency of fever and the use of intravenous antibiotics were lower in the probiotic group than in the placebo group. The administration of probiotics enhanced the growth of anaerobe bacteria in the gut. The authors concluded that *these data, although based on a limited number of patients and samples, suggest that administration of B. breve strain Yakult could be an effective approach for achieving clinical benefits in immunocompromised hosts by improving their intestinal environments.*[84]

A systematic review suggested that probiotics may reduce the severity and frequency of diarrhoea in patients with cancer and may reduce the requirement for anti-diarrhoeal medication, but more studies are needed to assess the true effect. The authors concluded that *probiotics may be a rare cause of sepsis.*

---

[84] Wada M, Nagata S, Saito M, Shimizu T, Yamashiro Y, Matsuki T, Asahara T, Nomoto K. Effects of the enteral administration of Bifidobacterium breve on patients undergoing chemotherapy for pediatric malignancies. Support Care Cancer. 2010 Jun;18(6):751–9. https://doi.org/10.1007/s00520-009-0711-6. Epub 2009 Aug 14. Erratum in: Support Care Cancer. 2010 Sep;18(9):1235–6. PMID: 19685085.

Further evidence needs to be collated to determine whether probiotics provide a significant overall benefit for people with cancer.[85]

A 2020 review of the clinical trial data stated that *the research results indicate, among others that peri-operative administration of probiotics effectively reduces postoperative infectious complications. Infection during abdominal surgery, which is considered a factor in patients' morbidity, can be reduced by administering probiotics to patients prior to surgery. In addition, it turns out that certain probiotic microorganisms are useful in the control of various intestinal disorders, including fever, postoperative inflammatory diseases, viral diarrhoea and antibiotic or chemotherapy/radiotherapy-associated diarrhoea.*[86]

And a 2021 review suggested that *probiotics may potentially be efficacious in reducing complications associated with chemotherapy, radiotherapy and surgery in patients with cancer.*[87]

The collective evidence thus suggests that probiotics might gain a place in palliative and supportive cancer care; however, at present it is not conclusive.

Plausibility	👍
Effectiveness	👎/👍
Safety	👍
Cost	👍
Risk/benefit balance	👎/👍

Propolis

Propolis or bee glue is the substance that bees produce by mixing their saliva with bee wax with exudate from tree buds, sap flows and other plant materials. Bees use it as a sealant for open spaces in the hive. Propolis is said to have

[85] Redman MG, Ward EJ, Phillips RS. The efficacy and safety of probiotics in people with cancer: a systematic review. Ann Oncol. 2014 Oct;25(10):1919–1929. https://doi.org/10.1093/ann onc/mdu106. Epub 2014 Mar 11. PMID: 24618152.

[86] Śliżewska K, Markowiak-Kopeć P, Śliżewska W. The Role of Probiotics in Cancer Prevention. Cancers (Basel). 2020 Dec 23;13(1):20. https://doi.org/10.3390/cancers13010020. PMID: 33374549; PMCID: PMC7793079.

[87] Miarons M, Roca M, Salvà F. The role of pro-, pre- and symbiotics in cancer: A systematic review. J Clin Pharm Ther. 2021 Feb;46(1):50–65. https://doi.org/10.1111/jcpt.13292. Epub 2020 Oct 23. PMID: 33095928.

several health benefits for humans, and it is available as a dietary supplement. In relation to cancer care, it is claimed to be effective against mucositis.

Oral mucositis is one of the most frequent complications after chemotherapy or radiotherapy or a combination of both. There is no standard therapy for its prevention or treatment. In a 2016 RCT with 40 cancer patients undergoing chemotherapy compared a propolis mouthwash to placebo. Oral mucositis, erythema and eating and drinking ability were assessed. There were significant differences in oral mucositis, wound and erythema in propolis group compared to placebo, but no significant difference in eating and drink ability. 65% of the patients in the propolis group were completely healed at day 7 of the trial. No significant adverse events were reported. The authors concluded that *oral care with propolis as mouthwash for patients undergoing chemotherapy is an effective intervention to improve oral health.*[88]

A 2018 systematic review included 5 RCTs with a total of 209 participants. The incidence of severe oral mucositis was significantly lower in the propolis group than in the control group. The authors concluded that *propolis mouthwash is effective and safe in the treatment of severe oral mucositis.*[89]

Thus, there is reasonably sound evidence that propolis can help cancer patients suffering from mucositis.

Plausibility	👍
Effectiveness	👍
Safety	👍
Cost	👎
Risk/benefit balance	👍

[88] AkhavanKarbassi MH, Yazdi MF, Ahadian H, SadrAbad MJ. Randomized DoubleBlind Placebo-Controlled Trial of Propolis for Oral Mucositis in Patients Receiving Chemotherapy for Head and Neck Cancer. Asian Pac J Cancer Prev. 2016;17(7):3611–4. PMID: 27510017.

[89] Kuo CC, Wang RH, Wang HH, Li CH. Meta-analysis of randomized controlled trials of the efficacy of propolis mouthwash in cancer therapy-induced oral mucositis. Support Care Cancer. 2018 Dec;26(12):4001–4009. https://doi.org/10.1007/s00520-018-4344-5. Epub 2018 Jul 19. PMID: 30022350.

Vitamin C

Vitamin C (Sect. 3.4) or ascorbic acid was first discovered in 1912. It is contained in numerous dietary supplements. Some studies have reported low plasma levels of vitamin C in cancer patients. Considering its many important functions, vitamin C is often recommended to cancer patients during supportive and palliative care.

To investigate the effects of vitamin C on cancer patients' health-related quality of life, Korean researchers gave 39 terminal cancer patients an intravenous administration of 10 g vitamin C twice with a 3-day interval and an oral intake of 4 g vitamin C daily for a week. Subsequently, their quality of life improved. The patients reported significantly higher scores for physical, role, emotional, and cognitive function after administration of vitamin C. The patients also reported significantly lower scores for fatigue, nausea/vomiting, pain, and appetite loss after administration of vitamin C.[90]

A 2014 review summarised three further prospective studies as well as case reports and retrospective studies indicating that intravenous (IV) vitamin C alleviates a number of cancer- and chemotherapy-related symptoms, such as fatigue, insomnia, loss of appetite, nausea, and pain. Improvements in physical, role, cognitive, emotional, and social functioning, as well as an improvement in overall health, were also observed.[91]

Controlled clinical trials of vitamin C as a treatment during palliative or supportive cancer care seem not to be available. Preliminary evidence suggests that vitamin C, both before and during breast cancer treatment, is associated with an increased risk of recurrence and death;[2] however, the evidence is contradictory.

Even though there is some suggestive evidence, it does not seem strong enough to justify the use of vitamin C in palliative or supportive cancer care.

Plausibility	👍
Effectiveness	✋
Safety	👍

(continued)

---

[90] Yeom CH, Jung GC, Song KJ. Changes of terminal cancer patients' health-related quality of life after high dose vitamin C administration. J Korean Med Sci. 2007 Feb;22(1):7–11. https://doi.org/10.3346/jkms.2007.22.1.7. PMID: 17297243; PMCID: PMC2693571.

[91] Carr AC, Vissers MC, Cook JS. The effect of intravenous vitamin C on cancer- and chemotherapy-related fatigue and quality of life. Front Oncol. 2014 Oct 16;4:283. https://doi.org/10.3389/fonc.2014.00283. PMID: 25360419; PMCID: PMC4199254.

(continued)

Cost	👍
Risk/benefit balance	👎

Vitamin E

Vitamin E was discovered in 1922 and is an umbrella term for a group of 8 fat-soluble antioxidants that include four tocopherols and four tocotrienols. It is contained in many oral and supplements and creams.

Topical vitamin E was shown to be beneficial in the treatment of oral mucositis in an RCT of patients with solid tumours or leukaemia. Six of 9 patients receiving vitamin E had complete resolution of oral lesions compared with 1 out of 9 in the control group.[92] In another study with 80 cancer patients with oral mucositis, 100 mg of a topical application of vitamin E was shown to improve mucositis.[93] In a further study with 54 patients with head and neck cancers, it was found that topical vitamin E reduced the risk of mucositis by 36%.[94] Finally, topical vitamin E and was shown in an RCT to reduce mucositis in 72 children.[95] Some but not all of the available evidence suggests that oral vitamin E supplementation might be associated with an increased risk of recurrence and death.[2]

On balance, the evidence is encouraging that topical vitamin E might be helpful in treating oral mucositis after cancer therapy.

Plausibility	👍
Effectiveness	👍

(continued)

[92] Wadleigh RG, Redman RS, Graham ML, Krasnow SH, Anderson A, Cohen MH. Vitamin E in the treatment of chemotherapy-induced mucositis. Am J Med. 1992 May;92(5):481–4. https://doi.org/10.1016/0002-9343(92)90744-v. PMID: 1580295.

[93] El-Housseiny AA, Saleh SM, El-Masry AA, Allam AA. The effectiveness of vitamin "E" in the treatment of oral mucositis in children receiving chemotherapy. J Clin Pediatr Dent. 2007 Spring;31(3):167–70. PMID: 17550040.

[94] Ferreira PR, Fleck JF, Diehl A, Barletta D, Braga-Filho A, Barletta A, Ilha L. Protective effect of alpha-tocopherol in head and neck cancer radiation-induced mucositis: a double-blind randomized trial. Head Neck. 2004 Apr;26(4):313–21. https://doi.org/10.1002/hed.10382. PMID: 15054734.

[95] Khurana H, Pandey RK, Saksena AK, Kumar A. An evaluation of Vitamin E and Pycnogenol in children suffering from oral mucositis during cancer chemotherapy. Oral Dis. 2013 Jul;19(5):456–64. https://doi.org/10.1111/odi.12024. Epub 2012 Oct 18. PMID: 23078515.

(continued)

Safety	👍
Cost	👍
Risk/benefit balance	👍

4.6 Paranormal Healing

Paranormal (or energy) healing is an umbrella term for a range of esoteric healing practices which are often poorly differentiated. Their common denominator is the belief in some form of mystical 'energy' that can be used for therapeutic purposes. Such practices have existed in many ancient cultures, and the 'New Age' movement has brought about a revival of these ideas. Today paranormal healing systems are amongst the most popular of all SCAMs.

The 'energy' referred to by such healers is distinct from the concept of energy in physics; it alludes to some life force such as chi in Traditional Chinese Medicine, prana in Ayurvedic medicine, or the vital force in homeopathy. In this chapter, I will discuss those forms of paranormal healing that are commonly used by cancer patients.

Crystal Healing

Crystal healing is the use of stones and crystals for medicinal purposes. Crystal therapists believe that specific crystals can emit specific healing energies and are capable of remembering both positive and negative events. Healing crystals, they allege, can thus be programmed and might, from time to time, need deleting unhelpful energies.[96] Many crystal therapists make very specific claims about specific crystals in the supportive care of cancer patients, e.g.:

---

[96] https://www.holisticshop.co.uk/articles/introduction-guide-crystals.

- Yellow Tiger Eyes: *This healing stone for cancer. It gives courage and strength to fight the disease. It is used as a healing crystal for lung cancer, lymphoma, and leukaemia.*
- Quartz *is a great crystal for cancer, it has the ability to absorb the negative energy from your chakra system. It then expels this bad energy into the ground. this is why quartz is such a great crystal to heal cancer.*
- Emerald: *This is a common skin cancer healing crystal so be sure to give this a try, if you are, unfortunately, facing skin cancer.*[97]

The assumptions of crystal healers fly in the face of science, and there is no evidence that the therapeutic claims made for crystal healing are true.

Plausibility	👎
Effectiveness	👎
Safety	👍
Cost	🤏
Risk/benefit balance	👎

Distant Healing

Distant healing is a form of paranormal healing where healers operate at often considerable distances from the patient. Proponents of distant healing do not consider distance to be a problem, as their 'healing energy' is not hindered by space. Healers send their 'healing energy' in the belief that it is received by the patient and thus stimulates her self-healing potential. The therapy is advocated for a wide range of conditions, including cancer.

There has been some research testing whether distant healing is effective. However, most of the studies available to date have serious methodological flaws; their findings are therefore not reliable. One review of 8 clinical trials showed that the majority of the rigorous trials do not support the hypothesis that distant healing has any specific therapeutic effects.[98] One RCT tested

---

[97] https://crystalopedia.com/crystals-for-cancer/.

[98] Ernst E. Distant healing--an "update" of a systematic review. Wien Klin Wochenschr. 2003 Apr 30;115(7–8):241–5. https://doi.org/10.1007/BF03040322. PMID: 12778776.

the effectiveness of distant healing for cancer. It did not provide evidence supporting its effectiveness.[99]

Plausibility	👎
Effectiveness	👎
Safety	👍
Cost	👍
Risk/benefit balance	👎

Faith Healing

Faith healing is a form of paranormal healing through divine intervention. The Bible and other religious texts provide numerous examples of divine healing, and believers consider them as a proof that faith healing is possible. There are also numerous reports of people suffering from severe diseases, including cancer, allegedly healed by divine interventions. A 2019 survey from France showed that 43% of pediatric cancer patients had used faith healing.[100]

Faith healing often takes the form of laying on hands where the preacher claims to channel the divine energy via his hands into the patient's body. Some places of pilgrimage, such as Lourdes in France, specialise in faith healing and produce seemingly impressive statistics. However, they do not withstand scientific scrutiny. A review of the 'cures' recorded in Lourdes showed that no significant effects have been certified during a 30 year

---

[99] Pagliaro G, Pandolfi P, Collina N, Frezza G, Brandes A, Galli M, Avventuroso FM, De Lisio S, Musti MA, Franceschi E, Esposti RD, Lombardo L, Cavallo G, Di Battista M, Rimondini S, Poggi R, Susini C, Renzi R, Marconi L. A Randomized Controlled Trial of Tong Len Meditation Practice in Cancer Patients: Evaluation of a Distant Psychological Healing Effect. Explore (NY). 2016 Jan-Feb;12(1):42–9. https://doi.org/10.1016/j.explore.2015.10.001. Epub 2015 Oct 26. PMID: 26657031.

[100] Menut V, Seigneur E, Gras Leguen C, Orbach D, Thebaud E. Utilisation des médecines complémentaires et alternatives chez l'enfant et l'adolescent atteint de cancer : une pratique fréquente [Complementary and alternative medicine use in two French pediatric oncology centers: A common practice]. Bull Cancer. 2019 Mar;106(3):189–200. French. https://doi.org/10.1016/j.bulcan.2018.11.017. Epub 2019 Feb 14. PMID: 30771881

period.[101] There is no evidence from rigorous clinical trials to show that faith healing is effective for palliative and supportive cancer care.

Plausibility	👎
Effectiveness	👎
Safety	👍
Cost	👍
Risk/benefit balance	👎

Pranic Healing

Pranic healing has ancient roots and was recently popularised by Choa Kok Sui (1954–2007). Pranic healers claim to stimulate the self-healing properties of our body. In Hinduism, prana is assumed to be the vital force that permeates the universe on all levels. Prana is believed to be the type of energy that is responsible for the body's health and maintenance. Prana is alleged to be essential for the body to function. Pranic healing is said to create and maintain health by restoring the energy of the chakras.

Pranic healing is often recommend as a treatment for cancer. There have been very few clinical trials of pranic healing. Those that have been published failed to porduce good evidence that it is effective for palliative or supportive cancer care.

Plausibility	👎
Effectiveness	👎
Safety	👍
Cost	👍
Risk/benefit balance	👎

---

[101] https://www.ncbi.nlm.nih.gov/pubmed/22843835.

Prayer

Prayer is amongst the oldest and most widespread interventions for alleviating illness and promoting good health. It is used by believers of all religions throughout the world. A US survey suggested that 72% of all US citizens pray for better health.[102] This makes prayer one of the most popular of all SCAMs.

Intercessory prayer is practised by people of all faiths and involves a person or group of persons setting aside time for petitioning God on behalf of another person. People who believe in the possibility that prayers might improve their health assume that God can be persuaded to intervene on their behalf by blessing them with healing energy.

Despite the lack of plausibility, numerous clinical trials of prayer have been conducted. Most of them fail to adequately control for bias, and their findings are mixed. A 2009 Cochrane review of all RCTs included 10 trials with a total of 7646 patients. The authors concluded *that the findings are equivocal and, although some of the results of individual studies suggest a positive effect of intercessory prayer, the majority do not and the evidence does not support a recommendation either in favour or against the use of intercessory prayer. We are not convinced that further trials of this intervention should be undertaken and would prefer to see any resources available for such a trial used to investigate other questions in health care.*[103] Since then, several further studies have been published.

- A 2012 RCT with 999 patients suffering from various cancers suggested that intercessory prayer generates *small but significant improvements in spiritual well-being.*[104]
- A 2020 RCT from Brazil included 31 breast cancer patients and found no relevant benefit of intercessory prayer when compared to a placebo control group.[105]

---

[102] Ross LE, Hall IJ, Fairley TL, Taylor YJ, Howard DL. Prayer and self-reported health among cancer survivors in the United States, National Health Interview Survey, 2002. J Altern Complement Med. 2008 Oct;14(8):931–8. https://doi.org/10.1089/acm.2007.0788. PMID: 18925865; PMCID: PMC3152800.

[103] Roberts L, Ahmed I, Hall S, Davison A. Intercessory prayer for the alleviation of ill health. Cochrane Database Syst Rev. 2009 Apr 15;2009(2):CD000368. https://doi.org/10.1002/14651858. CD000368.pub3. PMID: 19370557; PMCID: PMC7034220.

[104] Olver IN, Dutney A. A randomized, blinded study of the impact of intercessory prayer on spiritual well-being in patients with cancer. Altern Ther Health Med. 2012 Sep-Oct;18(5):18–27. PMID: 22894887.

[105] Miranda TPS, Caldeira S, de Oliveira HF, Iunes DH, Nogueira DA, Chaves ECL, de Carvalho EC. Intercessory Prayer on Spiritual Distress, Spiritual Coping, Anxiety, Depression and Salivary

The totality of the reliable evidence fails to show meaningful effects of prayer for palliative or supportive cancer care.

Plausibility	👎
Effectiveness	👎
Safety	👍
Cost	👍
Risk/benefit balance	👎

Reiki

Reiki is a form of paranormal healing popularised by Japanese Mikao Usui (1865–1926). It is based on the assumptions of Traditional Chinese Medicine and the existence of 'chi', the life force that is said to determine our health. Reiki practitioners believe that they can transfer 'healing energy' to a patient which, in turn, stimulates the flow of chi and the self-healing properties of the body. They assume that their healing power comes from the 'universal life energy' that provides strength, harmony, and balance to the body and mind.

Reiki is used for most conditions, including cancer. There have been several clinical trials testing the effectiveness of reiki. Unfortunately, their methodological quality is usually poor.

- A 2008 systematic review summarising this evidence concluded that *the evidence is insufficient to suggest that reiki is an effective treatment for any condition. Therefore, the value of reiki remains unproven.*[106]
- A 2019 systematic review was more optimistic and suggested that *Reiki therapy is useful for relieving pain, decreasing anxiety/depression and improving quality of life in several conditions. Due to the small number of studies in palliative care, we were unable to clearly identify the benefits of Reiki therapy, but preliminary results tend to show some positive effects of Reiki therapy for the end-of-life population. These results should encourage teams working in*

Amylase in Breast Cancer Patients During Radiotherapy: Randomized Clinical Trial. J Relig Health. 2020 Feb;59(1):365–380. https://doi.org/10.1007/s10943-019-00827-5. PMID: 31054062.

106 Lee MS, Pittler MH, Ernst E. Effects of reiki in clinical practice: a systematic review of randomised clinical trials. Int J Clin Pract. 2008 Jun;62(6):947–54. https://doi.org/10.1111/j.1742-1241.2008. 01729.x. Epub 2008 Apr 10. PMID: 18410352.

palliative care to conduct more studies to determine the benefits of Reiki therapy on pain, anxiety/depression and quality of life in palliative care.[107]

Only very few studies have tested the effectiveness of Reiki for cancer patients, and those that are available are far from rigorous. It would therefore be wrong to classify Reiki as an evidence-based therapy for cancer palliation and supportive care.

Plausibility	👎
Effectiveness	👎
Safety	👍
Cost	👍
Risk/benefit balance	👎

Spiritual Healing

Spiritual healing is similar to faith healing (see above), except that there is no need for the patient or the healer to believe in a deity. It has been defined as the direct interaction between the healer and a patient, with the intention of improving the patient's condition or curing the illness. Spiritual healers believe that the therapeutic effect results from the channelling of 'energy' from an undefined source into the patient. Their central claim is to promote or facilitate self-healing and well-being, both of which could be relevant to patients with cancer.

The evidence from clinical trials of spiritual healing is contradictory. Many clinical trials have serious flaws, and the most reliable studies fail to show effects beyond placebo. Research papers often fail to differentiate between different types of paranormal healing. One Cochrane review, for instance, found *inconclusive evidence that interventions with spiritual or religious components for adults in the terminal phase of a disease may or may not enhance well-being. Such interventions are under-evaluated. All five studies identified were undertaken in the same*

---

[107] Billot M, Daycard M, Wood C, Tchalla A. Reiki therapy for pain, anxiety and quality of life. BMJ Support Palliat Care. 2019 Dec;9(4):434–438. https://doi.org/10.1136/bmjspcare-2019-001775. Epub 2019 Apr 4. PMID: 30948444.

country, and in the multi-disciplinary palliative care interventions, it is unclear if all participants received support from a chaplain or a spiritual counsellor. Moreover, it is unclear in all the studies whether the participants in the comparative groups received spiritual or religious support, or both, as part of routine care or from elsewhere. The paucity of quality research indicates a need for more rigorous studies.[108]

Since the publication of this review, a further study has emerged. This Danish trial with 247 colorectal cancer patients found no positive effects. The authors' conclusions are clear: *Whereas it is generally assumed that ... healing has beneficial effects on well-being, our results indicated no overall effectiveness of energy healing on Quality of life, depressive symptoms, mood, and sleep quality in colorectal cancer patients.*[109]

Plausibility	👎
Effectiveness	👎
Safety	👍
Cost	👍
Risk/benefit balance	👎

Therapeutic Touch

Therapeutic touch (TT) is a form of paranormal healing developed by Dora Kunz (1904–1999), a psychic and SCAM practitioner, in collaboration with Dolores Krieger, a professor of nursing. TT is popular and practised predominantly by nurses. According to one TT-organisation, TT is *a holistic, evidence-based therapy that incorporates the intentional and compassionate use of universal energy to promote balance and well-being. It is a consciously directed process of energy exchange during which the practitioner uses the hands as a focus to facilitate the process.*[110] TT is used for most conditions, including cancer.

[108] Candy B, Jones L, Varagunam M, Speck P, Tookman A, King M. Spiritual and religious interventions for well-being of adults in the terminal phase of disease. Cochrane Database Syst Rev. 2012 May 16;(5):CD007544. https://doi.org/10.1002/14651858.CD007544.pub2. PMID: 22592721.

[109] Pedersen CG, Johannessen H, Hjelmborg JV, Zachariae R. Effectiveness of energy healing on Quality of Life: a pragmatic intervention trial in colorectal cancer patients. Complement Ther Med. 2014 Jun;22(3):463–72. https://doi.org/10.1016/j.ctim.2014.04.003. Epub 2014 May 2. PMID: 24906586.

[110] http://therapeutictouch.org/what-is-tt/.

Very few trials have tested TT on cancer patients.

- One RCT evaluated the effect of TT on pain-related parameters of in 90 male patients with cancer. Seven sessions of TT in 4 weeks were compared to a sham ritual (hands placed over the body as a gesture and moved without order) or standard care alone. The results suggested that *TT had a positive impact on the positive management of pain-related parameters in cancer patients. Therefore, TT is suggested to be used by healthcare providers as a complementary method for managing pain and its parameters.*[111]
- Another RCT included 90 cancer patients undergoing chemotherapy, exhibiting pain and fatigue of cancer. They were randomized to receive TT, sham-TT or usual care only. TT was more effective in decreasing pain and fatigue than the usual care group, while the placebo group indicated a decreasing trend in pain and fatigue scores compared with the usual care group.[112]
- Finally, another small RCT with breast cancer patients comparing TT with sham-TT suggested that *TT was effective in reducing vomiting in the intervention group.*[113]

All of these studies suffer from major weaknesses which render their findings less than reliable. Therefore, TT cannot be categorised as an evidence-based therapy for palliative and supportive cancer care.

Plausibility	👎
Effectiveness	👎
Safety	👍
Cost	👍

(continued)

[111] Tabatabaee A, Tafreshi MZ, Rassouli M, Aledavood SA, AlaviMajd H, Farahmand SK. EFFECT OF THERAPEUTIC TOUCH ON PAIN RELATED PARAMETERS IN PATIENTS WITH CANCER: A RANDOMIZED CLINICAL TRIAL. Mater Sociomed. 2016 Jun;28(3):220–3. https://doi.org/10.5455/msm.2016.28.220-223. Epub 2016 Jun 1. PMID: 27482166; PMCID: PMC4949034.

[112] Aghabati N, Mohammadi E, Pour Esmaiel Z. The effect of therapeutic touch on pain and fatigue of cancer patients undergoing chemotherapy. Evid Based Complement Alternat Med. 2010 Sep;7(3):375–81. https://doi.org/10.1093/ecam/nen006. Epub 2008 Feb 2. PMID: 18955319; PMCID: PMC2887328.

[113] Matourypour P, Vanaki Z, Zare Z, Mehrzad V, Dehghan M, Ranjbaran M. Investigating the effect of therapeutic touch on the intensity of acute chemotherapy-induced vomiting in breast cancer women under chemotherapy. Iran J Nurs Midwifery Res. 2016 May-Jun;21(3):255–60. https://doi.org/10.4103/1735-9066.180373. PMID: 27186202; PMCID: PMC4857659.

(continued)

Risk/benefit balance	

4.7   Other Forms of SCAM

Chiropractic

Chiropractic was created by Daniel David Palmer (1845–1913), an American magnetic healer who, in 1895, manipulated the neck of a deaf janitor allegedly curing the man's deafness. Palmer then promoted chiropractic as a cure-all and claimed that 95% of diseases were due to subluxations of spinal joints. The concept of spinal subluxations became the cornerstone of chiropractic 'philosophy'. Yet today we know that such subluxations do not exist.[114]

The evidence that spinal manipulation is effective beyond placebo is weak for back and neck pain and negative for all other conditions.[115] Many chiropractors claim to be able to help cancer patients. One website, for instance, states: *Chiropractic treatment can benefit cancer patients in many ways. It can reduce stress, increase mobility, and optimize function, and generally improve quality of life. By easing headaches and nausea, and relieving muscle tightness and neuropathy pain, chiropractic can help patients follow through with their treatment plans, which may even help extend their lives.*[116] Such statements are in sharp contrast to the published evidence which fails to show that chiropractic is effective for supportive or palliative cancer care.[117] Even some chiropractors have recently voiced concerns about misinterpretation of advertising any benefits for cancer patients from chiropractic care and acknowledged the lack of evidence in this area.[118]

---

[114] Mirtz TA, Morgan L, Wyatt LH, Greene L. An epidemiological examination of the subluxation construct using Hill's criteria of causation. Chiropr Osteopat. 2009 Dec 2;17:13. https://doi.org/10.1186/1746-1340-17-13. PMID: 19954544; PMCID: PMC3238291.

[115] Ernst E. Chiropractic: a critical evaluation. J Pain Symptom Manage. 2008 May;35(5):544–62. https://doi.org/10.1016/j.jpainsymman.2007.07.004. Epub 2008 Feb 14. PMID: 18280103.

[116] https://tuckclinic.com/blog/2017/03/30/cancer-and-chiropractic/.

[117] Alcantara J, Alcantara JD, Alcantara J. The chiropractic care of patients with cancer: a systematic review of the literature. Integr Cancer Ther. 2012 Dec;11(4):304–12. https://doi.org/10.1177/153 4735411403309. Epub 2011 Jun 10. PMID: 21665878.

[118] Laoudikou MT, McCarthy PW. Patients with cancer. Is there a role for chiropractic? J Can Chiropr Assoc. 2020 Apr;64(1):32–42. PMID: 32476666; PMCID: PMC7250516.

Spinal manipulation causes mild to moderate adverse effects, such as pain, in about 50% of all patients. In addition, it is associated with more serious complications, usually caused by neck manipulation damaging an artery that supplies parts of the brain resulting in a stroke and even death. Several hundred such cases have been documented in the medical literature—but, as there is no system in place to monitor such events, the true figure is almost certainly much larger.[119]

On balance, it seems clear that chiropractic can play no beneficial role in palliative and supportive cancer care.

Plausibility	👎
Effectiveness	👎
Safety	👎
Cost	👎
Risk/benefit balance	👎

Homeopathy

Homeopathy is based on principles that fly in the face of science (Sect. 3.2). Yet, it remains popular and to date around 500 clinical trials of homeopathy have been published. The totality of this evidence fails to show that homeopathic remedies are more than placebos.[120]

Yet, homeopathy is often promoted as an effective treatment for palliative or supportive cancer care. Our 2006 systematic review included 6 clinical trials. Their methodological quality was variable. We concluded that there was *insufficient evidence to support clinical efficacy of homeopathic therapy in cancer care.*[121] Since then, one remarkable further study has emerged. In this prospective, randomized, placebo-controlled, double-blind, three-arm,

---

[119] Stevinson C, Ernst E. Risks associated with spinal manipulation. Am J Med. 2002 May;112(7):566–71. https://doi.org/10.1016/s0002-9343(02)01068-9. PMID: 12015249.

[120] Ernst E. Homeopathy: what does the "best" evidence tell us? Med J Aust. 2010 Apr 19;192(8):458–60. PMID: 20402610.

[121] Milazzo S, Russell N, Ernst E. Efficacy of homeopathic therapy in cancer treatment. Eur J Cancer. 2006 Feb;42(3):282–9. https://doi.org/10.1016/j.ejca.2005.09.025. Epub 2006 Jan 11. PMID: 16376071.

multi-centre study, the researchers tested the effects of additive homeopathic treatment compared to placebo in patients with stage IV non-small cell lung cancer (NSCLC).

- 51 patients received individualised homeopathic remedies plus conventional treatments,
- 47 received placebo plus conventional treatments,
- 52 control patients without any homeopathic treatment were treated with conventional therapies and observed for survival only.

Quality of life (QoL) as well as functional and symptom scales showed significant improvement in the homeopathy group when compared with placebo after 9 and 18 weeks. Median survival time was significantly longer in the homeopathy group (435 days) versus placebo (257 days) as well as versus control (228 days). Survival rate in the homeopathy group differed significantly from placebo and from control. The authors concluded *that QoL improved significantly in the homeopathy group compared with placebo. In addition, survival was significantly longer in the homeopathy group versus placebo and control. A higher QoL might have contributed to the prolonged survival. The study suggests that homeopathy positively influences not only QoL but also survival.*[122] In view of the implausibility of homeopathy, these results are surprising and should be considered carefully. The first author is a well-known advocate of homeopathy, and it would be wise to wait for an independent replication before translating the findings into clinical practice.

Meanwhile, the totality of the reliable evidence does not show that homeopathy is an effective addition to palliative or supportive cancer care.

Plausibility	👎
Effectiveness	👎
Safety	👍
Cost	👍

(continued)

---

[122] Frass M, Lechleitner P, Gründling C, Pirker C, Grasmuk-Siegl E, Domayer J, Hochmayr M, Gaertner K, Duscheck C, Muchitsch I, Marosi C, Schumacher M, Zöchbauer-Müller S, Manchanda RK, Schrott A, Burghuber O. Homeopathic Treatment as an 'Add on' Therapy May Improve Quality of Life and Prolong Survival in Patients with Non-Small Cell Lung Cancer: A Prospective, Randomized, Placebo-Controlled, Double-Blind, Three-Arm, Multicenter Study. Oncologist. 2020 Oct 3. https://doi.org/10.1002/onco.13548. Epub ahead of print. PMID: 33010094.

(continued)

Risk/benefit balance	

Lakhovsky's Oscillator

George Lakhovsky believed that healthy cells emit radiation and, whenever a part of the body gets damaged, inflamed or ill, the resonance of those cells become less intense. When pathogenic bacteria or other microbes take over, they allegedly disrupt the functioning of healthy cells with their harmful frequency. Lakhovsky's oscillator is said to generate a field of frequencies in a broad spectrum. If a sick person is placed in this frequency spectrum, diseased cells are claimed to recognise their own frequency, tune in and start resonating in their own, healthy frequency again and the illness disappears.

The oscillator treatment thus aims at halting degenerative diseases like cancer. One website advertises the therapy as follows: *Have you lost a loved one to cancer? Georges Lakhovsky had a 98% success rate in treating fatal cancers over an 11-year period. Today we celebrate a 50% five-year survival rate.*[123]

Such claims are in sharp contrast with the published evidence which fails to show that Lakhovsky's oscillator is effective for cancer or any other condition.

Plausibility	👎
Effectiveness	👎
Safety	👍
Cost	👎
Risk/benefit balance	👎

Osteopathy

Osteopathy is a form of manual therapy invented over 100 years ago by the American Andrew Taylor Still (1828–1917). Today, US osteopaths (doctors of osteopathy or DOs) have more or less stopped practising manual therapy

---

[123] https://lakhovsky.com/.

and are fully recognised as medical doctors who can specialise in any medical field after their training which is similar to that of MDs. Outside the US, osteopaths practice almost exclusively manual treatments and are considered SCAM practitioners. Here we focus on the latter category of osteopaths.

Still defined his original osteopathy *as a science which consists of such exact, exhaustive, and verifiable knowledge of the structure and function of the human mechanism, anatomical, physiological and psychological, including the chemistry and physics of its known elements, as has made discoverable certain organic laws and remedial resources, within the body itself, by which nature under the scientific treatment peculiar to osteopathic practice, apart from all ordinary methods of extraneous, artificial, or medicinal stimulation, and in harmonious accord with its own mechanical principles, molecular activities, and metabolic processes, may recover from displacements, disorganizations, derangements, and consequent disease, and regained its normal equilibrium of form and function in health and strength.*[124]

Osteopathy is not dissimilar to chiropractic (see above). One important difference between the two disciplines is that osteopaths use less of those techniques which are associated with serious adverse effects. Osteopathy thus tends to be less harmful than chiropractic.

Some osteopaths consider themselves as back pain specialists, while others claim to effectively treat a much wider range of conditions, including cancer. Yet, hardly any reliable evidence has emerged to justify this. The aim of one Italian study was to assess the effect of osteopathic manipulation on pain relief and quality of life improvement in hospitalized cancer patients. A total of 23 patients were allocated to:

- the study group (OMT [osteopathic manipulative therapy] group, $N = 12$) who received osteopathic manipulative therapy (OMT) in addition to physiotherapy (PT),
- the control group (PT only, $N = 12$).

Pain and quality of life did not show any significant differences between the two treatments.[125]

There is thus no sound evidence to suggest that osteopathy has anything to offer to patients receiving palliative or supportive cancer care.

---

[124] http://www.gutenberg.org/ebooks/authors/search/?query=Still,+A.+T.+(Andrew+Taylor).

[125] Arienti C, Bosisio T, Ratti S, Miglioli R, Negrini S. Osteopathic Manipulative Treatment Effect on Pain Relief and Quality of Life in Oncology Geriatric Patients: A Nonrandomized Controlled Clinical Trial. Integr Cancer Ther. 2018 Dec;17(4):1163–1171. https://doi.org/10.1177/153473541 8796954. Epub 2018 Aug 31. PMID: 30168356; PMCID: PMC6247559.

Plausibility	👎
Effectiveness	👎
Safety	✋
Cost	👎
Risk/benefit balance	👎

Visceral Osteopathy

Visceral osteopathy (or visceral manipulation) involves the manual manipulation by a therapist of internal organs, blood vessels and nerves (the viscera) from outside the body. It was developed by the osteopath Jean-Piere Barral who claimed that, through his clinical work with thousands of patients, he created this modality based on organ-specific fascial mobilization.[126] According to its proponents, visceral manipulation is based on the specific placement of soft manual forces looking to encourage the normal mobility, tone and motion of the viscera and their connective tissues. These gentle manipulations are said to improve the functioning of individual organs, the systems the organs function within, and the structural integrity of the entire body.[127]

Visceral osteopathy is being practised mostly by osteopaths, less commonly by chiropractors and physiotherapists. It comprises of several different manual techniques firstly for diagnosing a health problem and secondly for treating it. Several studies have assessed the diagnostic reliability of the techniques involved. The totality of this evidence fails to show that they are sufficiently reliable to be of practical use.[128] Other studies have tested whether the therapeutic techniques used in visceral osteopathy are effective in curing disease or alleviating symptoms. The totality of this evidence fails to show that visceral osteopathy works for any condition.[14]

The aim of one study was to determine the impact of visceral osteopathy on the incidence of nausea/vomiting, constipation and overall quality of life (QoL) in women operated for breast cancer and undergoing adjuvant chemotherapy.

---

[126] https://www.barralinstitute.com/about/jean-pierre-barral.php.

[127] http://www.barralinstitute.co.uk/.

[128] https://bmccomplementalternmed.biomedcentral.com/articles/10.1186/s12906-018-2098-8.

Ninety-four women operated for a breast cancer stage 1–3, were randomly allocated to experimental or placebo group. Experimental group underwent a visceral osteopathic technique, while the placebo group was subjected to a superficial manipulation after each chemotherapy cycle. The results suggested that *osteopathy does not reduce the incidence of nausea/vomiting in women operated for breast cancer and undergoing adjuvant chemotherapy.*[129]

There is thus no sound evidence to suggest that visceral osteopathy is effective for palliative or supportive cancer care.

Plausibility	👎
Effectiveness	👎
Safety	👍
Cost	👍
Risk/benefit balance	👎

Yoga

Yoga is a system of healing that originates from ancient India. From the perspective of SCAM, it mainly includes gentle stretching exercises, breathing control, meditation and lifestyles (Fig. 4.3). The aim is to strengthen prana, the vital force as understood in traditional Indian medicine. Thus, it is claimed to be helpful for most conditions affecting mankind, including cancer.

There have been numerous clinical trials of various yoga techniques. They tend to suffer from poor study design and incomplete reporting. Their results are therefore not always reliable.

- A 2009 systematic review included 10 clinical trials. Its authors concluded that *although some positive results were noted, variability across studies and*

---

[129] Lagrange A, Decoux D, Briot N, Hennequin A, Coudert B, Desmoulins I, Bertaut A. Visceral osteopathic manipulative treatment reduces patient reported digestive toxicities induced by adjuvant chemotherapy in breast cancer: A randomized controlled clinical study. Eur J Obstet Gynecol Reprod Biol. 2019

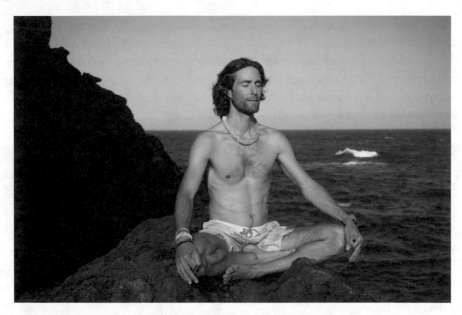

Fig. 4.3 Yoga combines physical exercises with meditation and life styles [*source Free Images on Unsplash*]

methodological drawbacks limit the extent to which yoga can be deemed effective for managing cancer-related symptoms.[130]

- A 2017 systematic review with 25 clinical trials concluded that *among adults undergoing cancer treatment, evidence supports recommending yoga for improving psychological outcomes, with potential for also improving physical symptoms. Evidence is insufficient to evaluate the efficacy of yoga in pediatric oncology.*[131]

- A 2017 Cochrane review included 24 studies and found that *moderate-quality evidence supports the recommendation of yoga as a supportive intervention for improving health-related quality of life and reducing fatigue and sleep disturbances when compared with no therapy, as well as for reducing depression, anxiety and fatigue, when compared with psychosocial/educational*

---

[130] Smith KB, Pukall CF. An evidence-based review of yoga as a complementary intervention for patients with cancer. Psychooncology. 2009 May;18(5):465–75. https://doi.org/10.1002/pon.1411. PMID: 18821529.

[131] Danhauer SC, Addington EL, Sohl SJ, Chaoul A, Cohen L. Review of yoga therapy during cancer treatment. Support Care Cancer. 2017 Apr;25(4):1357–1372. https://doi.org/10.1007/s00520-016-3556-9. Epub 2017 Jan 7. PMID: 28064385; PMCID: PMC5777241.

interventions. Very low-quality evidence suggests that yoga might be as effective as other exercise interventions and might be used as an alternative to other exercise programmes.[132]

Even though the evidence is full of contradictions, there is some encouraging evidence to suggest that yoga might be worth a try for patients in palliative or supportive cancer care.

Plausibility	👎
Effectiveness	👎 / 👍
Safety	👍
Cost	👍
Risk/benefit balance	👎 / 👍

[132] Cramer H, Lauche R, Klose P, Lange S, Langhorst J, Dobos GJ. Yoga for improving health-related quality of life, mental health and cancer-related symptoms in women diagnosed with breast cancer. Cochrane Database Syst Rev. 2017 Jan 3;1(1):CD010802. https://doi.org/10.1002/14651858.CD0 10802.pub2. PMID: 28045199; PMCID: PMC6465041.

5

Risks of SCAM

In the previous chapters, I have repeatedly mentioned the harms associated with the use of SCAM. The risks are obviously of prime importance; therefore, I will summarize the information in the following chapter.

For cancer patients, the following main risks need to be considered:

- The use of SCAMs as replacements for effective therapies
- The possibility that a SCAM is toxic
- Interactions between SCAMs and anti-cancer drugs.

5.1 SCAM as Replacements

Every cancer patient wants to receive the optimal therapy for their condition. One definition of the optimal treatment is a therapy that has the most favourable risk–benefit profile. Compared to the adverse effects of many conventional anti-cancer drugs, the risks of SCAM are usually small. This fact leads many practitioners of SCAM to claim that their options are preferable. However, as we have seen in Chap. 3, none of the SCAMs promoted as cancer cures are effective. This means that, even if their direct risks are relatively small, their risk–benefit balance is far from positive (Fig. 5.1).

Because none of the alternative cancer cures discussed in Chap. 3 are effective, the use of SCAM as a replacement of an effective therapy is never a good

E. Ernst, *So-Called Alternative Medicine (SCAM) for Cancer*,
https://doi.org/10.1007/978-3-030-74158-7_5

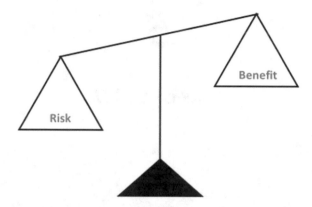

Fig. 5.1 The relationship between the risk and the benefit of a therapy can be explained by using the simple example of a scale: if a treatment conveys little or no benefit (small weight on the right arm of the scale), even relatively minor risks (weight on the left arm of the scale) will tilt the scale towards the left; conversely, if the benefits are huge, such as not dying of the disease, very considerable risks will be acceptable (this applies to many conventional treatments) [Copyright E Ernst]

idea. In fact, it is almost certain to significantly shorten the lives of cancer patients.

But the issue here is not necessarily one of 'all or nothing'; the use of SCAM has been shown to lower the adherence of cancer patients to their prescribed treatments. The objective of this study, for instance, was to investigate the relationship between the use of herbal remedies and medication adherence in elderly people. A random sample of Brazilian 240 elders was interviewed in their homes and the use of pharmaceutical medicines and of medicinal plants was assessed by direct examination. The results showed that medication non-adherence increased with use of herbal remedies, as well as with the number of different medicinal plants used. The authors concluded *that this study provides first-hand evidence that the use of herbal medicines is associated with poor medication adherence. Given the high frequency of the use of herbal medicines, further research into the mechanisms of this association is justified.*[1]

There is little doubt that employing SCAM in lieu of an effective treatment is the most serious danger associated with SCAM. It is for this reason that I repeated it throughout the book. In my view, one cannot warn patients and their carers often enough of it.

---

[1] Martins RR, Duarte Farias A, Russel Martins R, Gouveia Oliveira A. Influence of the use of medicinal plants in medication adherence in elderly people. Int J Clin Pract. 2016 Mar;70(3):254–60. http://doi.org/10.1111/ijcp.12773. Epub 2016 Jan 22. PMID: 26799730.

5.2 Toxic SCAMs

Cancer patients are continually bombarded with the notion that SCAM is harmless. Yet we have seen in the preceding chapters that this notion is not true, e.g.:

- Acupuncture can cause serious complications such as infections and injuries to vital organs.[2]
- Chiropractic spinal manipulations can cause arterial damage, followed by a stroke or even death.[3]
- Dietary supplements contain pharmacologically active ingredients which, depending on their nature, can cause all sorts of toxicities.[4]

Where they apply to specific SCAMs, these issues have been discussed in the respective chapters of this book. However, another problem has so far been neglected: the quality of SCAM preparations.

We need to be aware of the fact that SCAMs are not as stringently regulated as prescription drugs. Homeopathics, Bach flower remedies, Schuessler Salts, herbal remedies, non-herbal dietary supplements and other oral SCAMs are therefore not always of the quality one would expect of pharmaceuticals.

The issue has been studied best for herbal remedies. A systematic review, for example, aimed at summarising all available data relating to the heavy metal content in Indian herbal remedies. The results suggested that heavy metals, particularly lead, have been a regular constituent of traditional Indian remedies. This has repeatedly caused serious harm to patients taking such remedies. One study showed that 64% of samples collected in India contained significant amounts of lead (64% mercury, 41% arsenic and 9% cadmium).[5]

Equally concerning is the fact that Chinese herbal medicines (CHMs) are often adulterated. A systematic review summarized the data regarding adulterations of CHMs with conventional drugs. Eighteen case reports, two case

---

[2] Ernst E, Lee MS, Choi TY. Acupuncture: does it alleviate pain and are there serious risks? A review of reviews. Pain. 2011 Apr;152(4):755–764. http://doi.org/10.1016/j.pain.2010.11.004. PMID: 21440191.

[3] Stevinson C, Ernst E. Risks associated with spinal manipulation. Am J Med. 2002 May;112(7):566–71. http://doi.org/10.1016/s0002-9343(02)01068-9. PMID: 12015249.

[4] Ernst E. Risks of herbal medicinal products. Pharmacoepidemiol Drug Saf. 2004 Nov;13(11):767–71. http://doi.org/10.1002/pds.1014. PMID: 15386721.

[5] Ernst E. Heavy metals in traditional Indian remedies. Eur J Clin Pharmacol. 2002 Feb;57(12):891–6. http://doi.org/10.1007/s00228-001-0400-y. PMID: 11936709.

series and four analytical investigations were identified. The list of adulterants contains drugs associated with serious adverse effects like corticosteroids. In several instances, patients were seriously harmed. One report from Taiwan suggests that 24% of all samples were contaminated with at least one conventional pharmacological compound. It was concluded that *adulteration of CHMs with synthetic drugs is a potentially serious problem which needs to be addressed by adequate regulatory measures.*[6]

Such findings are concerning as they suggest that the quality of herbal and other dietary supplements is often substandard, even to the point where it endangers the health of the user. The best solution that I can offer to cancer patients is to be sceptical. If you feel you must use such products at all, it is advisable to purchase them from respectable suppliers.

5.3   Interactions Between SCAMs and Anti-cancer Drugs

If a cancer patient takes a SCAM product by mouth, and if that remedy has pharmacological effects, it is possible, even likely, that it will interact with other medications this patient is using concomitantly. Such interactions would have the following effects:

- They might increase the effects of the medication.
- They could decrease the effects of the medication.
- They might alleviate the side effects of the medication.
- They might aggravate the side effects of the medication.

In most cases, these interactions would be harmful and in almost all instances they would be unpredictable. An Australian Medicines Information Centre reviewed requests from cancer patients for information on interactions of 330 different SCAMs. The 10 SCAMs most commonly enquired about were fish oil (3.5%), turmeric (3.2%), coenzyme Q10 (2.6%), milk thistle (2.4%), green tea (2.4%), ginger (2.1%), lactobacillus (2.1%), licorice (1.8%), astragalus (1.8%) and reishi mushroom (1.6%). All were found

---

[6] Ernst E. Adulteration of Chinese herbal medicines with synthetic drugs: a systematic review. J Intern Med. 2002 Aug;252(2):107–13. http://doi.org/10.1046/j.1365-2796.2002.00999.x. PMID: 12190885.

to have predicted or potential drug interactions or therapeutic issues when combined with conventional therapies.[7]

We published a summary of all systematic reviews (SRs) of interactions between herbal medicinal products (HMPs) and synthetic drugs.[8] Forty-six SRs of 46 different HMPs met our inclusion criteria. The vast majority of SRs were of poor methodological quality. Serious herb–drug interactions were noted for St John's wort (*Hypericum perforatum*) and mistletoes (*Viscum album*). The most severe interactions resulted in:

- transplant rejection,
- delayed emergence from anaesthesia,
- cardiovascular collapse,
- renal and liver toxicity,
- cardiotoxicity,
- bradycardia,
- hypovolaemic shock,
- inflammatory reactions with organ fibrosis and death.

Moderately severe interactions were noted for Ginkgo biloba, Panax ginseng, Piper methysticum, Serenoa repens and Camellia sinensis (see Footnote 8). Dietary supplements that can interact with anti-cancer drugs include (see Footnote 5)[9] [10]:

- Antioxidants
- Cinnamon
- Black cohosh
- Echinacea
- Mistletoe
- Green tea

[7] Brooks SL, Rowan G, Michael M. Potential issues with complementary medicines commonly used in the cancer population: A retrospective review of a tertiary cancer center's experience. Asia Pac J Clin Oncol. 2018 Oct;14(5):e535–e542. http://doi.org/10.1111/ajco.13026. Epub 2018 Jun 22. PMID: 29932300.

[8] Posadzki P, Watson L, Ernst E. Herb-drug interactions: an overview of systematic reviews. Br J Clin Pharmacol. 2013 Mar;75(3):603–18. http://doi.org/10.1111/j.1365-2125.2012.04350.x. PMID: 22670731; PMCID: PMC3575928.

[9] Spagnuolo P. Interactions Between Nutraceutical Supplements and Standard Acute Myeloid Leukemia Chemotherapeutics. J Pharm Pharm Sci. 2015;18(4):339–43. http://doi.org/10.18433/j3m30k. PMID: 26626240.

[10] Yasueda A, Urushima H, Ito T. Efficacy and Interaction of Antioxidant Supplements as Adjuvant Therapy in Cancer Treatment: A Systematic Review. Integr Cancer Ther. 2016 Mar;15(1):17–39. http://doi.org/10.1177/1534735415610427. Epub 2015 Oct 26. PMID: 26503419; PMCID: PMC5736082.

- Noni
- Peppermint
- Red clover
- Saw palmetto
- Blessed thistle
- Reishi mushroom
- Senna
- St John's wort
- Turmeric
- Umckaloabo
- Zink.

In view of these facts, the notion often voiced by SCAM proponents that such SCAM-drug interactions are true rarities must be disavowed. A German study of 2016 assessed the frequency of interactions between SCAMs and drugs for comorbidities from a large survey on melanoma patients. Consecutive melanoma outpatients of seven skin cancer centres in Germany were asked to complete a questionnaire about SCAM-use and their medications for comorbidities and cancer. Each combination of conventional drugs and SCAMs was evaluated for their potential of interaction. A total of 1089 questionnaires were eligible for evaluation. From these, 62% of patients reported taking drugs regularly of whom 34% used SCAMs. Risk evaluation for interaction was possible for 180 SCAM users who listed the names or substances they took for comorbidities. Of those patients, 37% at risk of interaction of their co-consumption of conventional drugs and SCAMs. Almost all patients using Chinese herbs were at risk (89%).[11]

5.4　Conclusions

The inescapable conclusion from all this is that the three mantras of SCAM proponents.

- *SCAM is risk-free*
- *Conventional drugs cause harm*
- *SCAM is much safer than conventional medicine.*

---

[11] Loquai C, Dechent D, Garzarolli M, Kaatz M, Kaehler KC, Kurschat P, Meiss F, Stein A, Nashan D, Micke O, Muecke R, Muenstedt K, Stoll C, Schmidtmann I, Huebner J. Risk of interactions between complementary and alternative medicine and medication for comorbidities in patients with melanoma. Med Oncol. 2016 May;33(5):52. http://doi.org/10.1007/s12032-016-0764-6. Epub 2016 Apr 18. PMID: 27090799.

are naïve, ill-informed and at best the expression of wishful thinking. The truth is that SCAM can cause harm in multiple ways. In the interest of their health, cancer patients are well advised to heed this warning, be cautious and act wisely on the basis of robust evidence.

6

Conclusion

As we have seen in Chap. 3 of this book, there is no alternative cancer cure, nor will there ever be one. Yet, some might claim that, even though there is no single SCAM that cures cancer, the use of a tailor-made combination of SCAMs could be beneficial, particularly if employed in addition to conventional cancer treatments. In fact, we often hear claims that employing a package of diverse SCAMs can prolong the live or improve the quality of life of cancer patients. But are these assumptions true? While we have discusses specific SCAMs in the preceding chapters, I will now investigate whether a mixture of several SCAMs might prolong the life or improve the well-being of cancer patients.

Prolongation of Life

In 2003, a Norwegian study examined the association between SCAM-use and cancer survival. Of the 515 cancer patients included in the study, 112 had used SCAM. In total, 350 patients died during the 8 years of follow-up. Death rates were higher in SCAM users (79%) than in those patients who did not use SCAM (65%). The authors of this paper concluded that *the use of SCAM seems to predict a shorter survival from cancer.*[1]

---

[1] Risberg T, Vickers A, Bremnes RM, Wist EA, Kaasa S, Cassileth BR. Does use of alternative medicine predict survival from cancer? Eur J Cancer. 2003 Feb;39(3):372–7. http://doi.org/10.1016/s0959-8049(02)00701-3. PMID: 12565991.

© The Author(s), under exclusive license to Springer Nature Switzerland AG 2021
E. Ernst, *So-Called Alternative Medicine (SCAM) for Cancer*,
https://doi.org/10.1007/978-3-030-74158-7_6

In 2013, Korean researchers evaluated whether SCAM use affects the survival and health-related quality of life (HRQOL) of terminal cancer patients. They prospectively studied a cohort of 481 cancer patients. During a follow-up of 164 person-years, 466 patients died. Compared with non-users, SCAM users did not survive longer. The use of mind–body interventions (Sect. 4.3) or prayer (Sect. 4.6) was even associated with significantly worse survival. SCAM users reported significantly worse cognitive functioning and more fatigue than nonusers. In subgroup analyses, users of prayer, vitamin supplements, mushrooms, or rice and cereal reported significantly worse HRQOL. The authors conclude that *SCAM did not provide any definite survival benefit, CAM users reported clinically significant worse HRQOLs.*[2]

A 2017 study from Malaysia evaluated whether the use of SCAM among newly diagnosed breast cancer patients was associated with delays in presentation, diagnosis or treatment of breast cancer. A total of 340 newly diagnosed patients were included in this study. The authors found that *the use of SCAM was significantly associated with delay in presentation and resolution of diagnosis.*[3]

A 2017 US study was aimed at determining whether SCAM use impacts on the prognosis of breast cancer patients. A total of 707 patients with breast cancer completed a 30-month post-diagnosis interview including questions on SCAM use. During the observation period, 70 breast cancer-specific deaths and 149 total deaths were reported, and 60% of participants reported SCAM use post-diagnosis. No associations were observed between SCAM use and breast cancer-specific or total mortality. The authors concluded that *SCAM use was not associated with breast cancer-specific mortality or total mortality.*[4]

Another study included 281 patients with non-metastatic breast, prostate, lung, or colorectal cancer who chose SCAM, administered as sole anticancer

---

[2] Yun YH, Lee MK, Park SM, Kim YA, Lee WJ, Lee KS, Choi JS, Jung KH, Do YR, Kim SY, Heo DS, Kim HT, Park SR. Effect of complementary and alternative medicine on the survival and health-related quality of life among terminally ill cancer patients: a prospective cohort study. Ann Oncol. 2013 Feb;24(2):489–494. http://doi.org/10.1093/annonc/mds469. Epub 2012 Oct 30. PMID: 23110809.

[3] Mohd Mujar NM, Dahlui M, Emran NA, Abdul Hadi I, Wai YY, Arulanantham S, Hooi CC, Mohd Taib NA. Complementary and alternative medicine (CAM) use and delays in presentation and diagnosis of breast cancer patients in public hospitals in Malaysia. PLoS One. 2017 Apr 27;12(4):e0176394. http://doi.org/10.1371/journal.pone.0176394. PMID: 28448541; PMCID: PMC5407802.

[4] Neuhouser ML, Smith AW, George SM, Gibson JT, Baumgartner KB, Baumgartner R, Duggan C, Bernstein L, McTiernan A, Ballard R. Use of complementary and alternative medicine and breast cancer survival in the Health, Eating, Activity, and Lifestyle Study. Breast Cancer Res Treat. 2016 Dec;160(3):539–546. http://doi.org/10.1007/s10549-016-4010-x. Epub 2016 Oct 21. PMID: 27766453; PMCID: PMC5558457.

treatment. The results show that SCAM use was independently associated with greater risk of death compared with conventional cancer therapy (CCT). The authors concluded that *SCAM utilization for curable cancer without any CCT is associated with greater risk of death.*[5]

The same group of researchers compared overall survival of patients with cancer receiving CCT with or without SCAM. They used the National Cancer Database on 1,901,815 patients from 1500 Commission on Cancer-accredited centres across the US who were diagnosed with non-metastatic breast, prostate, lung, or colorectal cancer between January, 2004, and December, 2013. Patients were matched on age, clinical group stage, comorbidity, insurance type, race/ethnicity, year of diagnosis, and cancer type. The cohort included 1,901,815 patients with cancer, 258 patients in the SCAM group and 1,901,557 patients in the control group. The results showed that *patients who received SCAM were more likely to refuse additional CCT, and had a higher risk of death. The results suggest that mortality risk associated with SCAM was mediated by the refusal of CCT.*[6]

A 2020 analysis of the US National Health and Nutrition Examination Survey (NHANES) datasets (1999–2016) included a total of 4575 respondents with cancer. Among respondents with cancer, 3024 respondents reported the use of dietary supplements; while 1551 did not report the use of dietary supplements. The use of dietary supplements was not found to be associated with an advantage in overall survival.[7]

Finally, a 2021 study from Poland employed a survival analysis of cancer patients undergoing chemotherapy treatment with 42 months of follow-up time. The investigators found no statistical difference in overall survival between the groups that used and did not use any form of SCAM.[8]

Collectively, these studies do not demonstrate that SCAM use improves the prognosis of cancer patients. On the contrary, several investigations have suggested the opposite effect. There are, of course, several possibilities to explain why SCAM use might shorten the life of cancer patients, e.g.:

[5] Johnson SB, Park HS, Gross CP, Yu JB. Use of Alternative Medicine for Cancer and Its Impact on Survival. J Natl Cancer Inst. 2018 Jan 1;110(1). http://doi.org/10.1093/jnci/djx145. PMID: 28922780.

[6] Johnson SB, Park HS, Gross CP, Yu JB. Complementary Medicine, Refusal of Conventional Cancer Therapy, and Survival Among Patients With Curable Cancers. JAMA Oncol. 2018 Oct 1;4(10):1375–1381. http://doi.org/10.1001/jamaoncol.2018.2487. PMID: 30027204; PMCID: PMC6233773.

[7] Abdel-Rahman O. Dietary Supplements Use among Adults with Cancer in the United States: A Population-Based Study. Nutr Cancer. 2020 Sep 15:1–8. http://doi.org/10.1080/01635581.2020.1820050. Epub ahead of print. PMID: 32930008.

[8] Michalczyk K, Pawlik J, Czekawy I, Kozłowski M, Cymbaluk-Płoska A. Complementary Methods in Cancer Treatment-Cure or Curse? Int J Environ Res Public Health. 2021 Jan 5;18(1):356. http://doi.org/10.3390/ijerph18010356. PMID: 33466517; PMCID: PMC7796472.

- Some of the SCAMs in question might have a direct adverse effect on cancer progression, for instance, by being toxic or by interacting with conventional cancer drugs.
- Patients who choose to use SCAM might be more ill than those who do not employ it. The Malaysian study (see Footnote 3) quoted above suggests that this is a possibility. In several studies, however, this factor has been taken into account and is, therefore, an unlikely explanation.
- Patients who opt for SCAM might takes conventional cancer treatments less seriously or even shun them completely. Several of the above-cited studies suggest that this is a likely explanation.
- The above-cited studies are mostly observational by nature. This means that we cannot be sure about cause and effect. In other words, the data are not fully convincing and the results could merely be an artefact.

Whatever the explanation, the undeniable fact is that there is no good evidence to suggest that the use of a mixture of SCAMs improves the natural history of cancer.

Improvement of Quality of Life

In Chap. 4, we have seen that some forms of SCAM—by no means all—benefit cancer patients in multiple ways. Therefore, some SCAMs do help generate a better quality of life (QoL) for cancer patients in palliative or supportive care. This begs the question whether a tailor-made package of SCAMs (rather that a single specific SCAM) might be even of more benefit than a single SCAM.

The purposes of this 2005 study were to compare the QoL in SCAM users and non-SCAM users and to determine whether SCAM use improves QoL among 546 breast cancer patients during chemotherapy. A total of 71% of patients were identified as SCAM users. There was no significant difference in global health status scores or QoL between the two groups. The authors concluded that *there was no significant difference between users and non-users of SCAM in terms of QoL.*[9]

The aim of a 2019 study was to investigate the effects of a complex, nurse-led, supportive care intervention using SCAM on 126 cancer patients' QoL and associated patient-reported outcomes. Women with breast or gynae-cologic cancers undergoing chemotherapy (CHT) were randomly assigned

---

[9] Chui PL, Abdullah KL, Wong LP, Taib NA. Quality of Life in CAM and Non-CAM Users among Breast Cancer Patients during Chemotherapy in Malaysia. PLoS One. 2015 Oct 9;10(10):e0139952. http://doi.org/10.1371/journal.pone.0139952. PMID: 26451732; PMCID: PMC4599886.

to routine supportive care plus intervention (intervention group, IG) or routine care alone (control group, CG). The intervention consisted of SCAM applications and counselling for symptom management, as well as SCAM information material. No group effects on QoL were found upon completion of CHT, but there was a significant group difference in favour of the IG, 6 months later. IG patients did also experience significant better emotional functioning and less fatigue. The authors concluded that *the tested supportive intervention did not improve patients' QoL outcomes directly after CHT (T3), but was associated with significant QoL improvements when considering the change from baseline to the time point T4, which could be assessed 6 months after patients' completion of CHT. This delayed effect may have resulted due to a strengthening of patients' self-management competencies.*[10]

Confronted with conflicting results it is wise to see whether there are any good summaries of the totality of the evidence. A systematic review published in 2013 included 13 studies. Their findings were mixed, *either showing a significantly greater improvement in QoL in the intervention group compared to the control group, or no significant difference between groups.*[11]

A 2020 systematic review compared the effectiveness of SCAMs on the QoL of women with breast cancer. Twenty-eight clinical trials were included, 18 of which were randomised. The SCAM interventions included dietary supplements and a variety of mind–body techniques. Twenty-seven studies showed improved QoL. The authors concluded that *the findings may indicate the potential benefits of SCAMs, especially mind–body techniques on QOL in breast cancer patients.*[12]

These papers indicate four important points:

- The volume of the evidence for SCAM in palliative and supportive cancer care is currently by no means large.
- The primary studies are often methodologically weak and their findings are contradictory.

---

[10] Klafke N, Mahler C, von Hagens C, Uhlmann L, Bentner M, Schneeweiss A, Mueller A, Szecsenyi J, Joos S. The effects of an integrated supportive care intervention on quality of life outcomes in outpatients with breast and gynecologic cancer undergoing chemotherapy: Results from a randomized controlled trial. Cancer Med. 2019 Jul;8(8):3666–3676. http://doi.org/10.1002/cam4.2196. Epub 2019 May 21. PMID: 31115192; PMCID: PMC6639168.

[11] Shneerson C, Taskila T, Gale N, Greenfield S, Chen YF. The effect of complementary and alternative medicine on the quality of life of cancer survivors: a systematic review and meta-analyses. Complement Ther Med. 2013 Aug;21(4):417–29. http://doi.org/10.1016/j.ctim.2013.05.003. Epub 2013 Jun 3. PMID: 23876573.

[12] Nayeri ND, Bakhshi F, Khosravi A, Najafi Z. The Effect of Complementary and Alternative Medicines on Quality of Life in Patients with Breast Cancer: A Systematic Review. Indian J Palliat Care. 2020 Jan-Mar;26(1):95–104. http://doi.org/10.4103/IJPC.IJPC_183_19. Epub 2020 Jan 28. PMID: 32132792; PMCID: PMC7017686.

- Several forms of SCAM have the potential to be useful in palliative and supportive cancer care.
- Therefore, generalisations are problematic, and it is wise to go by the current best evidence as outlined in Chap. 4.

Final Thoughts

Yes, things tend to be complex, emotions often fly high in the realm of SCAM and patients can lose patience with science and scientists. Such situations provide a fertile ground for conspiracy theories to grow. Indeed, a 2014 study from the US found that belief in conspiracy theories is rife in SCAM.[13] The investigators presented consumers with 6 different conspiracy theories. The one that was most widely believed was about SCAM: THE FOOD AND DRUG ADMINISTRATION IS DELIBERATELY PREVENTING THE PUBLIC FROM GETTING NATURAL CURES FOR CANCER AND OTHER DISEASES BECAUSE OF PRESSURE FROM DRUG COMPANIES. A total of 37% agreed with this statement, 31% had no opinion on the matter, and just 32% disagreed with it. What is more, the belief in this particular conspiracy correlated positively with the usage of SCAM.

This seems to suggest that the world of SCAM is at least partly driven by the conviction that there is a sinister plot by the FDA or more generally speaking 'the establishment' that prevents people from benefiting from the wonders of SCAM.

With this book, I have tried to outline the existing evidence and demonstrated that such notions are unfounded. Yet, mistrust is undoubtedly a core element in SCAM. Mistrust generates a rejection of authoritative information. If voices of authority are negated due to mistrust, the resulting void sends cancer patients "down the rabbit hole" in search for answers from an increasingly "post-truth" SCAM.

To regenerate trust, we need to provide reliable data, teach critical thinking, and enable patients to comprehend the evidence. That is what I wanted to achieve with this book, and I repeatedly emphasised my main messages:

- evidence needs to be understood by everyone;
- alternative cancer cures are a dangerous myth;

---

[13] Oliver JE, Wood T. Medical conspiracy theories and health behaviors in the United States. JAMA Intern Med. 2014 May;174(5):817–8. http://doi.org/10.1001/jamainternmed.2014.190. PMID: 24638266.

- some forms of SCAM can be helpful in palliative and supportive cancer care;
- SCAM is rarely totally risk-free;
- critical thinking saves lives.

I sincerely hope that my book makes a contribution towards the health, well-being and common sense of its readers.

Acknowledgements I am grateful to Dr. Julian Money-Kyrle, retired consultant oncologist, for his constructive comments on Sect. 1.4 and to Richard Rasker for his corrections of and advice on the entire text.

Appendix A: A Short Guide for Making Informed Choices

In 2019, some of the most influential experts in medicine published a paper entitled 'Key concepts for making informed choices'.[1] Here I have adopted some of their ideas and modified them for the purpose of cancer patients. The result might serve as a guide to those struggling to find their way through the maze of SCAMs on offer.

GENERAL:

- Belief is no substitute for evidence.
- Correlation is not the same as causation.
- The treatments you employ are only one of several factors that determine the outcome.
- Assumptions about how a form of SCAM might work are not a reliable form of evidence.
- More data are not necessarily better data.
- Trust in one single source of information is ill-advised.
- Peer review and publication by a journal do not guarantee reliability; in particular, journals that specialise in SCAM have a poor track record.

---

[1] Aronson JK, Barends E, Boruch R, Brennan M, Chalmers I, Chislett J, Cunliffe-Jones P, Dahlgren A, Gaarder M, Haines A, Heneghan C, Matthews R, Maynard B, Oxman AD, Oxman M, Pullin A, Randall N, Roddam H, Schoonees A, Sharples J, Stewart R, Stott J, Tallis R, Thomas N, Vale L. Key concepts for making informed choices. Nature. 2019 Aug;572(7769):303–306. https://doi.org/10.1038/d41586-019-02407-9. PMID: 31406318.

CLAIMS:

- Cancer patients are bombarded with claims about the value of SCAM. It is important to remember: if it sounds too good to be true, it probably is.
- Check where a health claim comes from and what conflicts of interest might be involved. Generally speaking, claims from anyone earning their income from SCAM are less reliable than those from independent investigators or institutions.
- Claims about SCAMs should be supported by reliable evidence (Sect. 1.8).
- SCAMs are not entirely risk-free; be cautious about sources that claim otherwise.
- Large, dramatic effects are very rare in SCAM; those who claim otherwise are misleading you.
- The results of one single study considered in isolation can be misleading.
- SCAMs that have been used for decades are not necessarily effective or safe.
- Experiences or anecdotes are an unreliable basis for therapeutic claims.
- Opinions of experts, authorities, celebrities or other respected individuals are not a reliable basis for claims.

CLINICAL TRIALS:

- Studies should be designed to minimize the risk of biases and random errors (i.e. the play of chance).
- The people, groups or conditions being compared in clinical trials should be treated similarly, apart from the interventions being studied.
- Outcomes should be assessed using methods that have been shown to be reliable.
- Outcomes should be assessed in all (or nearly all) the patients enrolled in a study.
- Small studies might be misleading.

CHOICES:

- Choices depend on judgements about the problem, the relevance (applicability or transferability) of evidence available and the balance of expected benefits, harm and costs.
- Available evidence should be relevant.
- Choices should focus on important and well-documented effects of SCAMs.

- The circumstances in which the SCAM was tested should be similar to those of the patient making the choice.
- Expected pros should outweigh cons.
- Uncertainties about the effects of SCAMs should be taken into account.

Appendix B: Recommended Sources of Information

Most cancer patients go on the Internet to find information about SCAM. It is therefore worth remembering that the Internet can be a dangerous place. Much of the information on SCAM to be gleaned from the Internet is promotional, unreliable and potentially harmful. Here are a few sites that usually provide information that is more reliable than most of the millions of further websites on SCAM.

American Cancer society Complementary and Alternative Methods and Cancer.

CAM-CANCER Cam-Cancer | Cam-Cancer (cam-cancer.org).

Cancer Research UK Complementary and Alternative therapies | Cancer Research UK.

Cancer Society NZ What are complementary and alternative medicines? | Cancer Society NZ - Auckland / Northland (cancernz.org.nz).

Cochrane Collaboration Cochrane | Trusted evidence. Informed decisions. Better health.

Cancer and alternative therapies – Good Thinking Society.

NHS Complementary and alternative medicine - NHS (www.nhs.uk).

Macmillan Cancer Support Alternative therapies - Macmillan Cancer Support.

My own blog Edzard Ernst.

National Cancer Institute Complementary and Alternative Medicine (CAM) - National Cancer Institute.

E. Ernst, *So-Called Alternative Medicine (SCAM) for Cancer*, https://doi.org/10.1007/978-3-030-74158-7

Glossary

Abstract summary of a scientific paper.

Acupuncture therapy from China involving the insertion of needles into the skin and underlying tissues at special points for therapeutic or preventative purposes.

Adjuvant therapy a treatment administered in addition to other interventions.

Adverse effect unwanted side effect of a therapy.

Bias a systematic deviation from the truth. In research, bias is likely to produce results that are wrong or misleading.

Blinding a term used in controlled clinical trials to describe the fact that trial participants are masked as to the allocation of patients into experimental or control groups.

Cachexia condition characterized by skeletal muscle and adipose tissue loss, an imbalance in metabolic regulation, and reduced food intake that can affect patients with advanced cancers.

Case control study investigation where two groups of patients, one with and one without a defined characteristic, are compared.

Case report a document that includes all the relevant details of one single and typically remarkable clinical case.

Causality the principle that there is a cause for everything that happens.

Clinical outcome the term used for quantifying the results of clinical trials or studies.

Cochrane review a systematic review conducted according to the Cochrane methodology and published by the Cochrane Collaboration.

Compassion the feeling of sympathy and sadness for the suffering of others and a wish to help.

Conflict of interest a situation in which someone's personal interests are opposed to that person's responsibilities to other people.

© The Editor(s) (if applicable) and The Author(s), under exclusive
license to Springer Nature Switzerland AG 2021
E. Ernst, *So-Called Alternative Medicine (SCAM) for Cancer*,
https://doi.org/10.1007/978-3-030-74158-7

Control group the name of the group of patients in a controlled clinical trial receiving the treatment, often a placebo, to which the experimental therapy is being compared.

Controlled clinical trials a study where patients are divided into two or more groups receiving different interventions the effects of which are compared at the end of the treatment period.

Correlation relation between phenomena or variables which occur in a way not expected based on chance alone.

Critical thinking (assessment, evaluation) the process of conceptualizing, applying, analysing, synthesizing, and/or evaluating information gathered by observation, experience, reflection, reasoning, and/or communication.

Detoxification the term used in SCAM for treatments that allegedly eliminate toxins from the body; often shortened to 'detox'.

Double-blind the term used in clinical trials indicate that both the patient as well as the investigators do not know whether the patient has been allocated to the control or the experimental group.

Effectiveness (of a treatment) the clinical effects caused by the therapy (rather than by other phenomena such as the placebo effect) as demonstrated under real-life conditions.

Efficacy (of a treatment) the clinical effects caused by the therapy under strictly controlled conditions.

Empathy the awareness of the feelings and emotions of other people.

Energy the capacity to perform work, measured in units of Joules. Energy exists in several forms such as heat, kinetic or mechanical energy, light, potential energy, electrical energy. In SCAM, the term is often applied to a patient's vital force as postulated by proponents of the long-obsolete philosophy of vitalism.

Evidence the body of facts that leads to a given conclusion.

Evidence-based medicine (EBM) the integration of best research evidence with clinical expertise and patient values. EBM thus rests on three pillars: external evidence, ideally from systematic reviews, the clinician's experience, and the patient's preferences.

Experimental group the name of the group of patients in a clinical trial who receive the treatment that is being tested.

Fallacy a commonly used argument that appears to be logical but, in fact, is erroneous.

Hazard ratio the ratio of the hazard rates corresponding to the conditions described by two levels of an explanatory variable. For example, in a drug study, the treated group may die at twice the rate as the control group.

Hypothesis a proposed explanation for a phenomenon. To be scientific, a hypothesis ought to be testable. Hypotheses are usually based on observations that cannot be satisfactorily explained with the currently existing scientific theories.

Individualised treatment a therapy that is tailored not primarily to the diagnostic category but to the personal characteristics of a patient. homeopaths, traditional herbalists, and TCM practitioners individualise their treatments.

In vitro outside living organisms; for example, in a test tube.

In vivo in living organisms, for example, in a cell culture.

Lay practitioner a clinician who has not been to medical school.

Life force see vital energy

Medline the world largest electronic database of papers published in medical journals.

Meta-analysis a systematic review where the results of the included primary studies have been mathematically pooled to generate a new overall finding.

Mucositis painful inflammation of the mucous lining the digestive tract, often an adverse effect of chemotherapy and radiotherapy.

Multifactorial a term to describe a situation where multiple causes contribute to an observed effect or outcome.

Natural history of a disease the course of a condition when left untreated.

Nonspecific effect a determinant of the clinical outcome other than the effect of the applied treatment itself.

Observational study a non-experimental investigation, usually without a control group. In a typical observational study, patients receiving routine care are monitored as to the treatments administered and the outcomes observed.

Outcome measure the parameter or endpoint employed in clinical studies for quantifying their result or outcome, for instance, survival time or quality of life.

Panacea a therapy that allegedly is effective for every condition or disease.

Pilot study an investigation that is preliminary and typically aimed at determining whether a given protocol is feasible for testing a hypothesis.

Placebo a treatment that has no effects per se but can appear to be effective through the placebo effect which essentially is due to expectation and conditioning.

Plausibility logical explanations for an observed or postulated phenomenon. The plausibility of therapy depends on whether its mechanism of action can be understood in the light of accepted scientific facts.

Post-marketing surveillance the monitoring of adverse effects of therapy while it is used by millions of patients. In conventional medicine, it is usually achieved by a reporting scheme which notifies the regulator of all observed problems. In SCAM, no effective post-marketing surveillance systems are in place.

Quality of life the state of well-being of a person. It can be measured by various means (e. g. validated questionnaires such as the 'SF36') and used to monitor the success of SCAMs and other therapies. It is often employed as an outcome measure in clinical trials.

Randomisation means dividing the total group of participants of a clinical trial in typically two subgroups purely by chance, e. g. by throwing dice. The desired effect of randomisation is that the two subgroups are comparable in all known and even unknown characteristics.

Randomised clinical trial (RCT) a controlled clinical trial where patients are allocated to experimental or control groups by randomisation, e.g. relying on chance alone.

Regression towards the mean the phenomenon that, over time, extreme values or outliers tend to move towards less extreme values. Patients normally consult clinicians when they are in an extreme situation (e. g. when they have much pain).

Because of the regression towards the mean, they are likely to feel better the next time they visit. This change is regardless of the effects of any treatment they may have had. Regression towards the mean is therefore one of several phenomena that can make an ineffective therapy appear to be effective.

Relative risk the ratio of the probability of an outcome in an exposed group to the probability of an outcome in an unexposed group.

Risk factor a variable associated with an increased risk of a condition to occur.

Sample size the size of the group of individuals entered into a research study.

Science the identification, description, observation, experimental investigation, and theoretical explanation of phenomena.

Selection bias a situation where an analysis has been conducted among a subset of a sample with the goal of drawing conclusions about the entire sample; the resulting conclusions will likely be wrong (biased), because the subgroup differs from the population in some important way.

Sham a placebo intervention, for instance, a placebo treatment (sham acupuncture) mimicking real acupuncture.

Significance a term used in research in two different contexts. Statistical significance describes the likelihood by which a given research result is due to chance. Often it is expressed by providing a 'p-value', i. e. a measure of probability. A p-value of 0.05 indicating statistical significance means that chances are 5 in 100 that the result in question is due to chance. Clinical significance (or relevance) describes the likelihood by which a clinical result is important in a clinical context. For instance, a study might show that a homeopathic treatment has lowered systolic blood pressure by 3 mmHg; this could well be statistically significant but few experts would call it clinically significant.

Specific effect the effect caused by therapy per se, rather than by placebo or other non-specific effects.

Symptomatic treatment a treatment aimed at alleviating symptoms without treating the cause of the underlying condition.

Systematic review a critical evaluation of the totality of the available evidence related to a specific research question. Systematic reviews minimize the bias inherent in each single trial.

Theory the result of abstract thinking about generalized explanations of how nature works. A theory provides an explanatory framework for a set of observations. From the assumptions of the explanation follow several possible hypotheses that can be tested in order to provide evidence for or against the theory.

Vital energy a metaphysical concept of a power that allegedly animates all organisms.

Vitalism the metaphysical concept that life depends on vital energy or force distinct from chemical, physical or other scientifically principles. It is a concept found in many forms of SCAM, e. g. chi in China, pneuma in ancient Greece, and prana in India. The common denominator is the assumption that metaphysical energy animates all living systems.

Printed in the United States
by Baker & Taylor Publisher Services